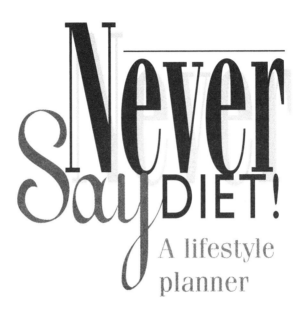

Never Say DIET!

A lifestyle planner

7 DAYS A WEEK

Judy Toews MSc, RDN
Nicole Parton
Illustrations by Graham Harrop

KEY PORTER BOOKS

Canadian Cataloguing in Publication Data

Toews, Judy, 1946–
    Never say diet...7 days a week

ISBN 0-55263-008-0

1. Reducing. 2. Food habits. 3. Women—Health and hygiene. 4. Diaries (blank books).
I. Parton, Nicole. II. Title.

RM222.3.T645 1998   613.2'5   C98-931398-0

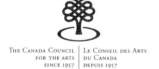

THE CANADA COUNCIL | LE CONSEIL DES ARTS
    FOR THE ARTS | DU CANADA
    SINCE 1957 | DEPUIS 1957

The publisher gratefully acknowledges the support of
the Canada Council for the Arts and the Ontario Arts
Council for its publishing program.

Key Porter Books Limited
70 The Esplanade
Toronto, Ontario
Canada M5E 1R2

www.keyporter.com

Design: Peter Maher
Electronic formatting: Heidy Lawrance Associates

Printed and bound in Canada

98 99 00 01 6 5 4 3 2 1

Note: The information in this book is for reference and education and is not intended to
take the place of a physician's advice. The publisher and authors disclaim any liability, loss,
or risk that is incurred as a consequence of the application of any of the contents of this book.

This is the first day of the rest of your life ...

Welcome to the first step on the journey toward a new, healthier you! This little lifestyle planner will guide you to guilt-free, delicious eating, active living, and peace of mind. Open it to today's date—and begin!

Don't wait until you're less busy or less tired. By gently focusing your attention on your needs, this book will help you boost your energy level and manage your "busy-ness."

Remember us? We're Judy Toews and Nicole Parton, the dietitian and the former dieter who wrote *Never Say Diet!* If you read our first book, you already know diets don't work. Over time, they lead to weight *gain*, not loss. In *Never Say Diet!* you learned how to find your healthy best weight. This day planner will help you stay there, motivating and inspiring you every day of the year through our 3 E's of healthy living: Eating, Exercise and Ease of mind.

Didn't read our first book? Too bad —but don't let that hold you back. *Never Say Diet ... 7 Days a Week!* encourages healthful living every day of the week, every month of the year. Think of this book as a box of chocolates—an array of bite-sized tidbits to tickle your fancy. Each day offers a new tip with a fresh slant on one of the 3 E's, or a reminder to keep practicing healthy living.

Each of the 3 E's is highlighted on the page opposite the daily tips. In logical sequence, we outline a step-by-step approach to personally satisfying Eating, Exercise, and Ease of mind. You can start to "never say diet" at any point, on any day, but you may want to skim the whole book before getting started. We'd particularly like you to read pages 6, 8, 10, 12, 14, 16, and 18 to see how to make this program work for you.

Doesn't it feel good to check something off on your "To Do" list? On each calendar day, you'll find a place to check the little things you do for your health and vitality. Did you forgo your usual doughnut and sink your teeth into a juicy orange? Take a short walk? Grab a minute to consciously relax? As you make small changes in your daily habits, check off each of the 3 E's on your day planner.

Use the space titled "Today" to remind yourself to do something just for you, each day. Loving and nurturing yourself is empowering—and health-promoting.

You may lose weight following the 3 E's, but we urge you to think of this little book as one about winning rather than "losing." This is your day planner, accepting and supporting you at any size, nurturing your inner and outer beauty, and helping you achieve your potential to be your very best.

Judy and Nicole

Before you read on...

Not everyone can or should lose weight—but everyone can benefit from becoming more nutrition-conscious and feeling greater vitality. We suggest you do two things before you start:

- Read the Physical Activity Readiness Questionnaire (PAR-Q) on page 127, before becoming more physically active.
- If you're under medical care, discuss this program with your doctor before making any lifestyle changes. This book has been written for healthy, non-pregnant adults.

In these pages, we regularly recommend that you drink lots of water. For most people, that's good advice —but if you have a medical condition requiring fluid restriction (heart or kidney problems, for example), check with your doctor before increasing your water intake.

To all our readers, past and present:
Thank you for sharing the journey.

Diets Don't Work!

Ever felt you'd "failed" by falling off your diet? *You* didn't fail—your diet did. Diets make you fatter. That's a scientific fact. They not only slow down your metabolism, but they also set you up for failure with illogical, expensive, or ridiculously restrictive food combinations that leave you ravenous. Ever thought you could achieve a healthy best weight *and* feel vitally alive by eating amply and well? Read on!

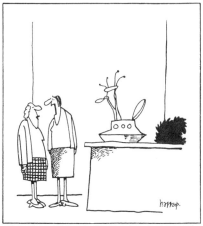

I'M GOING WITH THEM—THEY SAY I'D WEIGH ONLY 22 POUNDS ON THEIR PLANET...

The 3 E's of Healthy Living

You're about to discover 3 E-sy Basics that could change your life. Check each of the 3 E's on your daily lifestyle planner three times a day, as you:

 Eat with awareness

 Exercise briskly

 Ease conscious relaxation into your life

Start by dividing your day into three parts: morning, afternoon, and evening. During each, do the following:

• Eating: Replace one of your usual food or drink items with a more nutritious one—a bagel instead of a doughnut, or an apple instead of apple pie.
• Exercise: Move your body for one minute.
• Ease: Consciously relax for 30 seconds.

So far, so E-sy!

The Shape You're in Means More than Your Shape

Sizism starts at home. Kids hear their moms criticize their own normal adult bodies; TV sends repetitive signals that you've got to be "thin" to be smart, popular, well-dressed, glamorous, or "cool." Our obsession with weight has led to an upsurge in eating disorders that can lead to malnutrition, fertility problems, premature osteoporosis, or even death. Your fitness and health have more to do with your daily habits than with the numbers on your scale. Whether or not you lose weight, the 3 E's can boost your energy level and lower your risk of illness. *Never Say Diet ... 7 Days a Week!* will take you on a guided journey of self-discovery, one day at a time.

Binge Buster:	Make a "fresh" start today, eating one extra fruit or veggie at every meal. Color your first meals of the new year healthy!	🍐	👟	♡
Today:			**1**	
Goal Getter:	Keep a journal of daily positive thoughts that will send your motivation levels soaring. Write on!	🍐	👟	♡
Today:			**2**	
Moving Moment:	Walking is the world's oldest mass-transit system. It takes you out of yourself and away from your problems.	🍐	👟	♡
Today:			**3**	
Stats Quo:	Americans eat more on Super Bowl Sunday than on any other day of the year except Thanksgiving Day.	🍐	👟	♡
Today:			**4**	
Go with the Flow:	Sip a glass of water several times a day. Being dry can make you think you're hungry.	🍐	👟	♡
Today:			**5**	
Soul Provider:	Hold hands around the table. The food before you is the product of nature's bounty and others' labor. Give thanks.	🍐	👟	♡
Today:			**6**	
Incredible Edible:	Armchair athletes thrive on pretzels, air-popped corn, and raw veggies. Serve with plenty of chilled sparkling water.	🍐	👟	♡
Today:			**7**	

Beauty and the Best: Laughter grounds us in the present—there are no thoughts of yesterday or plans for tomorrow in that instant burst of joy.

The Journey and the Destination Are One

Got a pencil handy? The most important words in this lifestyle planner are the ones you will write yourself. That's why you'll find space for Notes to Myself throughout this little book. And that's why you *won't* find height–weight tables, calorie charts, or ready-made exercise plans.

If you're not happy with your weight now, this day planner will help you change either your weight or the way you feel about it. You'll learn a lot about yourself by writing down your thoughts. You're on a voyage of self-discovery to find the weight that's right for you.

It's your journey, but we'll be asking you questions—*personal ones*—to help you clarify your goals and plan for success. Make this a *private* day planner so you can feel totally free to be honest with yourself. Don't be tempted to skip the Notes to Myself section! It's guided, personal research that could very well change your life.

Old habits are comfortable because they let us do things without thinking. New, more positive habits take time and practice—but they're worth it! This lifestyle planner will *do* more than help you reshape your body. It will help you reshape your life and your future —at any size, at any age. You're on your way!

Mind Over Fatter

You may lose a few pounds at the start of any weight-loss diet, but your body soon adjusts to conserve every calorie. That means you eat less but weigh the same—or even more!

Focus on your health, energy, and vitality rather than a number on the scale. Plenty of thin people are out of shape—and plenty of full-figured people are fit. Achieving your healthy best weight is part of the process of becoming healthy—not just the goal.

Notes to Myself

How *would* I feel today if I had been eating well, exercising regularly, and relaxing daily for the past six months? How *do* I feel today?

Herb 'n' Renewal: *Today:*	Sprinkle on some fresh cilantro, dill, or basil instead of salt. Salt is a silent thief, robbing your bones of precious calcium.	🍐	👟	♡ **8**
Goal Getter: *Today:*	Change how your body feels before trying to change how it looks. Change on the inside produces change on the outside.	🍐	👟	♡ **9**
Incredible Edible: *Today:*	Stuff a baked potato with ricotta cheese for a low-fat, high-fiber treat. Or top that spud with salsa, lemon, or herbs.	🍐	👟	♡ **10**
Hello to Good Buys: *Today:*	Dried beans, lentils, and chick peas cost only a fraction of their canned equivalents. They're fiber and flavor bargains!	🍐	👟	♡ **11**
Stats Quo: *Today:*	Living dolls? If Barbie were a real woman, her measurements would be 36-18-33. She would also be seven feet tall. Go figure!	🍐	👟	♡ **12**
Soul Provider: *Today:*	Practice positive self-talk. If you think you can do it, you'll try! If you know you can do it, you will!	🍐	👟	♡ **13**
Twist and Pout: *Today:*	Prevent exercise injuries by warming up at the start, and cooling down at the end, with gentle stretching and mild activity.	🍐	👟	♡ **14**

Beauty and the Best: You can't control how long you live, but you can control how well you live.

Choosing Vitality

The impulse that made you pick up this book sprang from wanting to be the best you can be. Pause a moment to think about what that means. Maybe you'd like to lose weight. More importantly, what do you want to gain? Confidence? Power? Respect? Energy? Fitness? Strength? Peace of mind? These and other qualities are linked with health and vitality. Weight loss may or may not be part of the picture.

We can't predict the future, but we can plan opportunities for ourselves. Life doesn't offer guarantees—but it does offer daily choices. By practicing the 3 E's, you're choosing vitality. Let this lifestyle planner help your motivation soar!

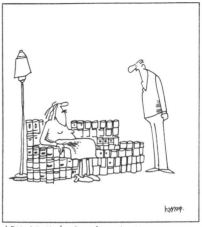

I REPEAT – YOU'RE BECOMING OBSESSED WITH FOOD…

Facing Change

Everything in the world, from fragile blossoms to rock-solid mountains, undergoes constant change. Every cell in our bodies is regularly renewed.

Because it means stepping outside the comfort zone of familiar routines, changing the way we eat or exercise can be scary. Doubts can arise like big black clouds, making us want to run for the shelter of old habits.

Counter doubts with positive self-talk. And then let the doubts go. Your body experiences change every second of your life. Why not put yourself in the driver's seat and steer your own course?

Notes to Myself

Why do I want to change my weight? How do I want to feel about myself after I've done so?

Poultry in Motion: *Today:*	Doing nothing more than removing the skin from a serving of dark-meat chicken legs trims 10 grams—or 90 calories—of fat!	🍐 👟 ♡ **15**
Goal Getter: *Today:*	People who like people are more stress-resistant. Those with many social ties are less susceptible to the common cold.	🍐 👟 ♡ **16**
Moving Moment: *Today:*	Make your exercise "routine" less routine and more fun. Vary it as you do your food. Skip, hop, jump—be playful!	🍐 👟 ♡ **17**
Stats Quo: *Today:*	Three-quarters of women consider nutrition important, while only slightly more than half of men surveyed feel the same way.	🍐 👟 ♡ **18**
Go with the Flow: *Today:*	Spritz it up and drink it down. Dilute wine or fruit juice with an equal amount of soda water. Full taste! Half the calories!	🍐 👟 ♡ **19**
Soul Provider: *Today:*	Stretch your limbs. Stretch your mind. Stretch your outlook!	🍐 👟 ♡ **20**
Full Lives: *Today:*	No time for a workout? Try 10-minute mini-movers—weights in the morning, a walk at lunch, an exercise video at night.	🍐 👟 ♡ **21**

Beauty and the Best: Life's banquet offers many and varied pleasures—indulge your senses by fully experiencing what each day offers.

11

Weigh to Go!
The Living Is E-sy!

Perhaps you weigh more than you think you should, but aren't ready to make a change. That's okay. That's not an excuse, but reality. Change made too fast doesn't last. When you feel ready to change, you'll know it.

While carrying too much weight can be linked to medical conditions such as diabetes, hypertension, heart attacks, or certain types of cancer, it's not always unhealthy to be a little above average in weight. People with very high or very low weights are at greatest risk for health problems.

You may be at your healthy best weight right now. If so, great! Here's an opportunity to enhance your fitness and well-being, while feeling in control of your weight. No need to shed pounds if you're already there!

Some people decide to lose weight on a whim. They set an arbitrary number and call it their "goal." What could be more self-defeating than working toward the wrong goal?

If you want to become more positive, energetic, and bursting with vitality, this book's for you. The 3 E's of healthy living can help you reach that goal on a daily basis, regardless of your long-term plans.

Notes to Myself

What personal strengths do I have? How can these qualities help me manage my weight?

Moving Moment: *Today:*	Reading fitness-oriented books and magazines will pump you up about shaping up. They're major motivators for a healthy lifestyle.			**22**
Goal Getter: *Today:*	Most women consider exercise important to health, but few exercise regularly. Physical activity never used to be considered "feminine," but those days are gone!			**23**
In Bod We Trust: *Today:*	Elderly tomboys? Older women who were active as girls are more likely to be active today. Their bodies want to move!			**24**
Stats Quo: *Today:*	The salt we sprinkle on food is only five percent of our intake. The rest comes from prepared foods—frozen meals, salad dressings, sauces, snacks, and condiments.			**25**
Soul Provider: *Today:*	The healthiest women don't cling to youth. They focus on qualities that improve with age —experience, maturity, wisdom.			**26**
The Light Stuff: *Today:*	Many pita and tortilla "wraps"—even the vegetarian ones—are higher in fat and calories than they look. Split one with a friend.			**27**
Binge Buster: *Today:*	Allowing yourself an occasional treat will help keep you on track in finding your healthy best weight. Bon appetit!			**28**

Beauty and the Best: Imagine your spirit floating free, just outside your body. Focus on your breathing, deep and slow. Let your spirit slip back into your body. You are happy, serene, content.

Which Weight Is Best?

How much should you weigh? You're probably the best person to answer that question. Your body is yours alone. You're unique!

One measure of healthy best weight is the Body Mass Index (BMI), an internationally accepted guide for people 19 to 60 years old. See the instructions below to calculate yours. A BMI of 20 to 25 is often referred to as a "healthy weight" range, although some medical and nutritional scientists put the upper limit at 30 or more, especially for older people.

The BMI is only a guide. You may feel more comfortable skipping the math, if you have a "usual" or natural weight you've maintained for several years. If you're 50 or older, being a little heavier than you were in your 20s may be appropriate. If you're muscular, your best weight may be higher than average, since muscle weighs more than fat. If you inherited a stocky build or a tendency to gain weight easily, your "genes" may always be snug! If you've had an above average weight for many years, or repeatedly gained and then lost pounds, it may be harder for you to lose weight than it is for some people.

Do you have a pretty realistic idea of a good personal weight, based on experience and the information we've given you? If not, ask your doctor to refer you to a dietitian and take this book along. If you do decide to lose weight, aim for an average weekly loss of about a pound (450 grams). If you lose too much too fast, you'll just gain it back. You may already know that from experience!

If you have a physical disability that makes it hard to exercise, you may find it difficult to lose excess fat. Use the exercises your physical therapist approves, rather than those we suggest.

The Body Mass Index: Guiding Your Goals

To determine your BMI, multiply your weight in pounds by 703, then divide the result by the square of your height in inches. For example, if you weigh 142 pounds and are 5'4" (64") tall, your BMI is (142 x 703) divided by (64 x 64), or 99,826 divided by 4,096, which equals 24.4. If you use the metric system, divide your weight in kilograms by the square of your height in meters.

Notes to Myself

My present weight is _____. My estimated healthy best weight is _____.

To get there, my weight change will be _____.

The approximate date for reaching my personal best weight is _____.

Stats Quo:	The U.S. food industry spends nearly $40 billion a year on advertising—most of it intended to make people eat more, rather than better.			29
Today:				
The Light Stuff:	Instead of cream cheese or sour cream, enjoy yogurt cheese! Pour plain, natural yogurt into a colander lined with a coffee filter, dripping it into a bowl, and chill overnight. Delicious!			30
Today:				
Binge Buster:	Read potato-chip and corn-chip labels. A "serving" could be as few as 15 chips! Count your portion before snacking—then put the bag away.			31
Today:				

Beauty and the Best: You make a living by what you get. You make a life by what you give.

From Apples to Pears

Are you an apple or a pear?

If extra weight settles in your lower body, you're pear-shaped. The bad news: Fat around the lower body is more stable than fat around the middle, making it harder to lose. The good news: Extra weight around the lower body isn't linked to any health hazard.

If extra weight settles around the middle of your body, you're apple-shaped. The bad news: Abdominal fat gets into the bloodstream with ease, increasing the risk of diabetes and heart disease. The good news: It's easier to lose fat from the middle of your body than fat from your lower body.

Men who put on weight tend to be apple-shaped, and women, pear-shaped.

Hip, Hip, Hooray!

Healthy bodies come in all sizes, shapes, and weights. Your waist–hip ratio is a good indicator of the healthiness of your body shape. It lets you know when you lose fat around the middle, even if your weight stays the same. Pear-shaped folks look better if their upper bodies aren't too thin, so they may not want to lose too much weight. If you can't decide if you're an apple or a pear, you may be some of each!

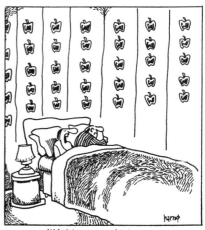

I'M HUNGRY AGAIN...

Notes to Myself

For women, health risk is lowest at waist–hip ratios of 0.7 or less, and highest at 0.9 or more. For men, health risk is lowest at waist–hip ratios of 0.8 or less, and highest at 1.00 or more.

At the narrowest part, my waist is _____.

At the broadest part, my hips are _____.

Dividing my waist measurement by my hip measurement, my waist–hip ratio is

_____.

16

Binge Buster: *Today:*	"Fast" equals "fat"? Not with dried pasta, canned lentils and beans, tortillas, fresh and frozen veggies, and tofu on hand.			**1**
Goal Getter: *Today:*	Instead of dining properly, about a third of us snack two or more times a week at supper-time. When you snack, have three "real" foods and make it a mini-meal.			**2**
Second Helpings: *Today:*	Beef up a meatless spaghetti sauce with veggies. Mushrooms, celery, onions, and grated carrot all work well with tomato sauce.			**3**
Stats Quo: *Today:*	Ever "eaten like a bird"? A woman would have to consume 134 pounds (61 kilograms) of food each day to actually do so!			**4**
Waist Not, Want Not: *Today:*	Caution! One jumbo muffin easily equals four minis. Try a mini-muffin instead of a regular one.			**5**
Soul Provider: *Today:*	Life happens even when you don't pay attention. Be mindful. Every "ordinary" day offers extraordinary moments.			**6**
Moving Moment: *Today:*	Because it's a weight-bearing exercise, walking helps prevent osteoporosis. Strength training can make your bones even stronger!			**7**

Beauty and the Best: Studies show that if you walk 20 to 30 minutes or take part in a low-impact aerobics session several times a week and at least three hours before bedtime, you'll fall asleep faster and sleep better than sedentary folk.

Appetite for Life

At least some of the time, most of us use food as a reward, a friend, a pacifier—a source of comfort, fun, and delight. Eating should mean pleasure and joy, not guilt and fear.

It's normal to eat when you're hungry and stop when you're satisfied. But it's also normal to eat too much or too little, now and then.

Many of us eat because it's "meal time," whether we're hungry or not. If we don't know when we're hungry, how can we know when we've had enough? Others ignore hunger for hours, and then eat too fast or too much. Still others deny themselves food in satisfying quantities, and are always famished.

Enjoying food while finding and maintaining the weight that's best for you is a learned skill. *How* you eat can be as important as *what* you eat. You're about to discover your skill power—a new way of paying attention to your body's inner wisdom, so you will when you're hungry and when you're satisfied.

Leaving Normal

Do you feel "fat" when others say you're not? Do you stuff yourself and then feel the urge to vomit? Do you sometimes eat all the time, and find it hard to stop? If so, you could have an eating disorder. Call your public health department to find out who you can talk to. You *deserve* to feel comfortable about food and about your body.

Reminder!

- Eat with awareness!
- Exercise briskly!
- Ease conscious relaxation into your life!

Notes to Myself

Now that I've firmed up my goal, I'll record how I feel about my body, today.

Month	Weight/ BMI	Waist	Hips	Waist–Hip Ratio	Feelings About Myself
Month 1					
Month 2					
Month 3					
Month 4					
Month 5					
Month 6					

Goal Getter:	Tuna canned in oil has more than 10 times as much fat as tuna canned in water! Even if you rinse it off, oil-packed tuna has substantially more fat than water-packed tuna.	🍐	👟	♡
Today:			**8**	
A Leg Up:	Researchers say treadmills are the best machines for aerobic activity and fat-burning —better than stair-climbers, rowing machines, or stationary bikes.	🍐	👟	♡
Today:			**9**	
Skill Power:	Veggies and fruit are great health protectors—the more colorful, the better! Choose five to ten each day.	🍐	👟	♡
Today:			**10**	
Heavy Breathing:	Get a friend, get a dog, get a life! For motivation to get moving, buddy up! It may be easier to hit the pavement with a pal.	🍐	👟	♡
Today:			**11**	
Binge Buster:	Scuttle a snack attack. Stocking only healthy snacks—like apples or unbuttered popcorn —lessens high-fat cravings.	🍐	👟	♡
Today:			**12**	
Soul Provider:	Take a low-fat cooking class. Buy some workout duds. Renewing your motivation helps you renew yourself.	🍐	👟	♡
Today:			**13**	
Stats Quo:	About 340 million pairs of athletic shoes were sold in the U.S. last year. That's 1.3 pairs per person. Are you wearing yours?	🍐	👟	♡
Today:			**14**	

Beauty and the Best: There is magic in every moonbeam that bathes us in its light. Dance with the elves! Polish the stars! Anything is possible when you let your mind run free.

Refine Your Style

The Art of Eating

Stay tuned! The Art of Eating will guide you to:

- Refine your eating style
- Eat early and eat often
- Gauge your intake
- Make your calories count
- Practice power snacking

your attention from how your body feels. It's like being on automatic pilot—you're not really "there."

When you don't eat with awareness, it's easier to lose track of how much and how often you eat. Eating with awareness takes practice!

The Hunger Exercise

It's time to make some bigger changes. You've already replaced one of your usual food or drink choices with a more nutritious item three times a day. Changing some of what you eat is a great start! Now let's look at how you eat. Your inner wisdom can help you recognize hunger and satiety (the feeling that you've had sufficient food). Outer distractions—boredom, fatigue, stress, eating on the run, or eating in front of the TV—weaken inner wisdom, because they divert

Design Your Plan

Choose a time of the day when you're especially likely to eat for non-hunger reasons. Instead of snacking, wait until you're hungry—at least three hours (but not more than five) from your last meal.

Eat something enjoyable and nourishing that you can store for future use if you don't finish.

Sit down, eating the food very slowly. Pause frequently, trying to notice if you're starting to feel satisfied. Try to stop just when you feel satisfied. If you're hungry a little while later, permit yourself to have more.

Notes to Myself

For 24 hours, I will notice what prompts me to eat. In a non-judgmental way, I'll ask myself if I was truly hungry when I ate and if I stopped when I was satisfied.

Date/ Time	Food/Amount	Reasons for Eating: Hunger? Other? (specify)	Reasons for Stopping: Satiety? Other? (specify)

Moving *Moment:*	In-line skating puts much less stress on the body than running—if you don't take an unprotected tumble! Wear a helmet as well as wrist, elbow, and knee pads.			**15**
Today:				

Sylph *Esteem:*	A well-rounded life doesn't mean changing your dress size, but it may mean changing your lifestyle.			**16**
Today:				

Soul *Provider:*	Stress can trigger up to 1,500 chemical changes in the brain and body, increasing your risk of disease. Add conscious relaxation to your busy schedule.			**17**
Today:				

Binge *Buster:*	Give yourself permission to enjoy special treats—but set a limit *before* you start eating. Then stick to it!			**18**
Today:				

Hello to *Good Buys:*	Shop smart. Write a list. Shop *after* you've eaten. Let others buy their own treats. And avoid the aisle of capricious snacks!			**19**
Today:				

Goal *Getter:*	Believe in yourself: An optimistic outlook will keep you from sabotaging your goal of reaching your healthy best weight.			**20**
Today:				

Dine-o- *Mite:*	Forget oil-based marinades! Brush foods to be grilled or broiled with a mixture of mustard powder, garlic, a shot of soy sauce, and enough water to make a paste.			**21**
Today:				

Beauty and the Best: Worrying about the future will not change it. Set a time limit for mulling over problems. Do what you can today—then move on.

Create the Right Space

It's easier to notice and respond to hunger if you minimize outer distractions by eating in appropriate places and giving meals and snacks your full attention. That means not eating in your car, at your desk, or in front of the TV. Create the right space as you:

- Choose a new place to eat. If you already eat at a table, pick a new place and make it attractive. Light a candle. Enjoy some restful music. Use placemats or a tablecloth. Make meals special, whether you eat alone or with others. Choose an away-from-home eating place, too. Try to eat only at your designated places.
- Eat slowly, to maximize your enjoyment. Notice when you start to feel satisfied.
- Remove "trigger" foods that tempt you to eat on automatic pilot. Buy only enough for one dessert or snack—and make it a quality choice.
- Plan enjoyable activities for times when you usually snack.
- Don't always eat alone. If possible, plan ahead what you'll eat and how. Relax before starting to eat.
- Remember to take short breaks partway through the meal—stop eating and enjoy the conversation.

Brain Food

It takes 20 minutes for your brain to get the message that your stomach has had enough. Eating too fast usually means overeating, because that message arrives too late.

The Passionate Peach

Eating is a sensuous experience. Let one finger smooth the circumference of a warm, sun-ripened peach. Notice how its rosy blush blends to gold and cream. Let your lips and tongue caress its downy skin. Let your teeth puncture its flesh. Feel its juice ooze through your fingers and dribble down your chin. Inhale its perfume. Prolong the pleasure with tiny bites.

Notes to Myself

Places I eat or drink (e.g., kitchen, office, car):

Activities that trigger my eating (e.g., watching TV, spectator sports):

Situations that trigger my eating (e.g., noisy kids, being near certain foods):

Conditions that make me feel comfortable with food:

Conditions that make me feel uncomfortable with food:

Skinny Dipping:	When fresh food is unavailable, choose frozen produce, or canned fruits packed in water rather than sugar syrup.	🍐	👟	♡
Today:			**22**	
Stats Quo:	About one third of women and 10 percent of men who are already at healthy weights still strive to slim down. What's wrong with this picture?	🍐	👟	♡
Today:			**23**	
Moving Moment:	Organize to exercise. Keeping fitness togs and equipment in one place increases the likelihood of action.	🍐	👟	♡
Today:			**24**	
Goal Getter:	Need help to slow down your eating? Rest your fork on your plate after every few mouthfuls, pausing to enjoy your surroundings or focus on a conversation.	🍐	👟	♡
Today:			**25**	
Go with the Flow:	Water is the elixir of life, necessary for transporting vitamins, minerals, and other nutrients to every part of your body.	🍐	👟	♡
Today:			**26**	
Nothing to Lose:	Smile and accept compliments graciously. People who welcome and believe praise are more likely to stick to lifestyle changes. Give yourself a back pat, too!	🍐	👟	♡
Today:			**27**	
Incredible Edible:	Popcorn is a healthy, high-fiber snack—but skip the butter. Add 1/4 cup (60 milliliters) of raw kernels to a top-folded paper bag. Microwave for two minutes on "high"—that's all it takes.	🍐	👟	♡
Today:			**28**	
Pace Maker:	Bonus day this year? Give yourself a bonus. Drop a few items from the list of things you "should" do—you deserve a break!	🍐	👟	♡
Today:			**29**	

Beauty and the Best: Hoping things change "tomorrow" rarely makes it happen. Trying to change them today is what matters.

Put Yourself in the Picture

Ready ... set ... go!

Have you started to eat with awareness more often? If not, why not? This is the time to remove any hurdles in your way.

Move beyond the 3 E-sy Basics (page 6) and check your day planner's **Eating icon** each day that you:

- Eat with awareness
- Separate eating from other activities
- Eat in appropriate places
- Savor your food

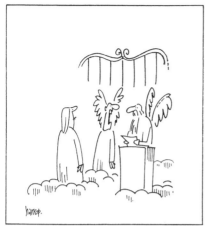

harrop.

SHE WANTS TO KNOW IF SHE CAN GO BACK FOR A BOX OF DOUGHNUTS SHE HID BEHIND THE FRIDGE ...

Taste Test Coming Up!

Practice your restaurant smarts! Ask a friend out to dinner, focusing on the skills you've learned so far. Or host a potluck in your kitchen. Combining food, friends, and fun enriches our lives.

Did You Know?

Nearly half of us eat in our cars at least once a week. More than half of us eat in front of the TV at least sometimes.

Notes to Myself

I visualize myself eating well and with awareness. How does it feel to be the person in that picture?

MARCH

Go with the Flow: Alcohol and caffeine are diuretics that increase your fluid losses. For every drink containing these little thieves, toss back a glass of water. **1** *Today:*		
Goal Getter: Read all about it! Brushing up on weight-control tips and smart eating practices is a strong motivator to keep your efforts on track. **2** *Today:*		
Moving Moment: Dust off those dumbbells. Resistance training tones and strengthens your body and turns back the hands of time. **3** *Today:*		
Skill Power: Spinach pasta doesn't contain much spinach. To boost your nutrient intake, toss small vegetable pieces into the pasta pot for the last three minutes of cooking. **4** *Today:*		
Discomfort Zone: People sometimes feel "bigger" than they are. Women can help each other determine if their body image is in sync with reality. **5** *Today:*		
Soul Provider: Laughter stimulates brain chemicals that prompt feelings of joy, stress reduction, and pain release. Positive thinking has physical benefits! **6** *Today:*		
Poultry in Motion: Skinned light-meat poultry has less fat and fewer calories than skinned dark meat. **7** *Today:*		

Beauty and the Best: Just for a moment, focus on one of your senses. Inhale the aroma of freshly baked bread. Smell wet grass. Sniff the pungent drift of wood smoke and reflect on the warmth of its fire.

Eat Early and Eat Often

Fuel Consumption

We give points for frequent eaters! Four to six small meals a day make it easier to manage your weight than three large meals.

Your body's metabolism—the rate at which you burn calories—slows down when you don't eat. Your body takes in fewer calories, but stores more of them as fat.

Regular eating teaches your body to expect a steady source of fuel. Your body doesn't need to become efficient at storing fat because it knows you will soon eat again. This is why some people seem to eat all the time while staying slim.

Fasting—going without food for long periods of time—makes you so hungry that when you finally eat, it's hard to know when to stop. Your body already fasts when you sleep. "Breaking the fast" with breakfast can help you control your weight.

The Hungry I

Skipping meals won't help you lose weight. People who skip breakfast and/or lunch often eat too much at night. Unfortunately, that's when your metabolism is at its lowest—it's the worst time to overeat. Weight lost when you fast is also easily regained.

There's more: Studies show that meal skippers tend to eat more high-fat foods than those who eat regular meals and a variety of foods.

Telling yourself you "won't eat" is useless—physiology always wins over psychology! We all have to eat to survive.

Notes to Myself

Am I eating well, taking the time for meals and snacks? What obstacles stand in my way? Which of my personal strengths can overcome them?

Leaps and Bounds:	Think about slotting exercise into a specific time each day—call it a date with yourself —and you'll make it a priority.	🍐	👟	♡
Today:			**8**	

Nothing to Lose:	Controlling your portions means your portions won't control you. Be mindful of what goes into your mouth.	🍐	👟	♡
Today:			**9**	

Moving Moment:	No time to exercise? Take three brisk 10-minute walks rather than a 30-minute walk.	🍐	👟	♡
Today:			**10**	

Stats Quo:	Afraid to quit smoking in case you gain weight? Most quitters gain no more than 10 pounds (4.5 kilograms). Many people who continue to smoke also gain weight.	🍐	👟	♡
Today:			**11**	

Goal Getter:	Don't give up baking for your health. Replace some of the butter or oil in recipes with prune or banana puree. Cut sugar amounts in half. Make desserts with a graham cracker crust instead of pastry.	🍐	👟	♡
Today:			**12**	

Soul Provider:	Ease helps prevent dis-ease! Practice two or three minutes of slow breathing at least three times a day.	🍐	👟	♡
Today:			**13**	

Binge Buster:	Watch those "social" drinks. Calorie-laden alcohol stimulates your appetite while affect ing your judgment. Plan ahead how much to drink. Stand by your plan!	🍐	👟	♡
Today:			**14**	

Beauty and the Best: Nurture your inner child. Give her room to grow in your heart, and the freedom to play in your soul.

Design Your Plan

Eat four to six times each day—three meals plus one to three light snacks, or six mini meals. Regular eating programs the brain to send your body the right signals for hunger and satiety, drawing on your body's inner wisdom. Try to eat regularly every day, and try to plan *when* to eat, too.

If you're not on track, use the Regular Eating Plan section below to make a new plan, spreading your eating evenly through the day and shifting some foods from meals to between-meal snacks. What you eat will change from day to day, but you can still use your new plan as a daily model.

Big Snack Attack

You can snack! We'll put the spotlight on power snacking just a little later.

Put Yourself in the Picture

Ready ... set ... go!

- When will you start your plan?
- What might interfere with it?
- How will you overcome obstacles, if any arise?

Check your day planner's **Eating icon** each day you spread your eating fairly evenly over the day, having about half your daily total by the time you've finished lunch.

Notes to Myself

I visualize myself eating regularly—never feeling too hungry or too full.

REGULAR EATING PLAN	
Morning Meal	**Morning Snack**
Midday Meal	**Afternoon Snack**
Evening Meal	**Evening Snack**

Incredible Edible:	Try broccoflower—a cross between broccoli and cauliflower. It packs more nutrients than cauliflower and, like broccoli, is a good source of vitamin C and beta-carotene.	🍐	👟	♡
Today:				**15**

Skinny Dipping:	Substitute low-fat buttermilk for the oil or cream in salad dressings, or for the butter and cream in mashed potatoes.	🍐	👟	♡
Today:				**16**

Go with the Flow:	Studies show that two glasses of plain, cold water arrest hunger better than a can of sugared pop.	🍐	👟	♡
Today:				**17**

Soul Provider:	To do simple things carefully and well is to become one with nature's harmony.	🍐	👟	♡
Today:				**18**

Mind Over Fatter:	Fat fattens! An ounce of fat has twice as many calories as an ounce of protein or carbohydrate. Fat on your lips means fat on your hips.	🍐	👟	♡
Today:				**19**

Skill Power:	Rinse canned fruit in cold water to wash away sugar syrup, and rinse fried ground beef in hot water to wash away excess fat.	🍐	👟	♡
Today:				**20**

Rites of Spring:	Weeding the garden, cleaning out the attic, scrubbing floors, and washing windows are more than spring cleaning—they're toners and firmers! Even moderate exercise burns calories.	🍐	👟	♡
Today:				**21**

Beauty and the Best: Appreciate what you have today, instead of wanting more tomorrow. It's never too late to give thanks. Count your blessings and be glad!

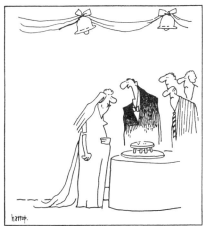

haref.

I THINK THE WEDDING CAKE WAS FOR EVERYBODY...

More than 90 percent of families feel it's important to share mealtimes as often as possible, and that meals are a time to socialize and communicate.

Boning Up on Fashion

The average North American woman stands 64 inches (163 centimeters) tall and weighs 140 pounds (63 kilograms). The average North American fashion model stands 70 inches (178 centimeters) tall and weighs 110 pounds (50 kilograms). Let's get real about lives and livelihoods!

Did You Know?

What foods do restaurant diners eat most? French fries lead the hit parade, followed by salad, pizza, bread, hamburgers, sweet baked goods, sandwiches, dessert, ice cream, and soup.
   What do they drink most? Coffee, soft drinks, tea, juice, beer, milk, wine, decaf coffee, and shakes.

Boning Up on Reality

Being too thin increases your risk of osteoporosis, or weak bones. Thirty percent of women and 15 percent of men suffer a hip fracture by age 90. About a third of them are institutionalized after the experience.

Notes to Myself

Eating isn't just about nutrition. What else is important to me in making food choices?

Leaps and Bounds:	It takes three months to become moderately fit, and six to get into shape. This small time investment will pay big health returns!			
Today:				**22**

Incredible Edible:	Add pureed vegetables to thicken tomato sauce, and you'll also boost the sauce's fiber.			
Today:				**23**

Poultry in Motion:	Don't let chicken à la king become chicken à la king-size! One serving of boneless chicken fits in the palm of your hand—it's the size of a deck of cards.			
Today:				**24**

Dine-o-Mite:	Show your restaurant smarts. Ask for veggies steamed without butter or sauce, and milk instead of cream for your coffee or tea.			
Today:				**25**

Stats Quo:	Many of us underestimate our daily food consumption by as much as 30 percent. Writing down what, when, and why we eat helps focus attention on quantity and quality.			
Today:				**26**

Moving Moment:	Try "retro" running or walking if your knees get sore. Moving backward eases the pressure. A forward-walking partner can pace you and help you stay safe.			
Today:				**27**

Goal Getter:	Reorganize to prioritize. If your favorite TV show interferes with your exercise time slot, videotape it for later viewing.			
Today:				**28**

Beauty and the Best: The greatest gifts are the sun, the moon, and the stars. Let them light up your world.

Gauge Your Intake

Many weight-conscious people don't eat enough to nourish their bodies. Canada's food guide (which combines vegetables and fruit) has four food groups. The food guides used in the U.S. and Australia (which consider vegetables and fruit separately) have five. These four or five food groups meet most people's nutrient needs. We've included Canada's daily recommended range of servings for adults beside each food group:

- Grain Products—carbohydrates, iron, B vitamins, and fiber (5-12 servings).
- Vegetables and Fruit—vitamin C, beta-carotene and other antioxidants, and fiber (5-10 servings).
- Milk and Alternatives—calcium, protein, and riboflavin (2 servings —4 if pregnant or nursing).
- Meat and Alternatives—iron, protein, and B vitamins (2-3 servings. We suggest a maximum of one from an animal source).

Foods high in sugar or fat and low in other nutrients don't rate a place in a food group. For that reason, they're sometimes known as "Other Foods." Use them sparingly!

How Much Is Enough —But Not Too Much?

A "serving" is easier to visualize using this handy guide:

- One serving of cheese or peanut butter is about the size of a pair of 3/4 inch (2 centimeter) dice.
- One serving of meat, fish, or poultry resembles a deck of cards.
- One medium apple, orange, or potato is about the size of a tennis ball.
- One cup (250 milliliters) of anything fills a regular-sized coffee mug; half a cup (125 milliliters) fills a dainty teacup.
- One serving of salad dressing, mayonnaise, or sour cream looks like two pats of butter.

Notes to Myself

How do the amounts you eat compare with the amounts in the sections above? Consider both numbers and sizes of servings.

☐ I'm eating larger-than-recommended amounts of food.
   Gradually start to cut back on foods you overeat, except for plain vegetables. Keep eating four to six times daily, but in smaller amounts.

☐ I'm eating moderate amounts at meals, but my snacks are too big.
   Gradually cut back on snack portions. More about snacking later!

☐ I'm eating moderate amounts, period.
   Your eating may need only fine-tuning. Exercise is likely your key to weight control.

☐ I'm eating a very low-calorie diet—much less than recommended.
   Don't cut back any further! You'll be able to gradually increase the amount you eat as you become more active.

Soul Provider:	Chinese wisdom: "When you are busy, your heart is dead. When you are relaxed, beauty reveals itself."		
Today:			29
Goal Getter:	Some researchers suggest that prolonged TV watching lowers your resting metabolic rate, making it easier to add unwanted pounds.		
Today:			30
Moving Moment:	Step up the pace. Swap 30 minutes of TV watching for 30 minutes of brisk walking. It's literally the time of your life.		
Today:			31

Beauty and the Best: Tackle one task at a time, setting realistic deadlines so you're busy but not stressed. Learning to say "no" means knowing your limits—and sticking to them.

Less Is Not Always Better

Be aware of eating too little. Your weight may stay the same and your general health may decline. Instead of eating less, you can eat more food by shifting from high-fat to low-fat, high-fiber foods.

- If you eat less than the amounts recommended last week, you may not be meeting your nutrient requirements.
- If you eat more grains, vegetables, and fruit than the minimum recommended for adults, that's not necessarily excessive. The higher your activity level, the more of these foods you'll need.
- On the other hand, extra servings of meat, milk products, and "Other Foods" can boost your fat intake.

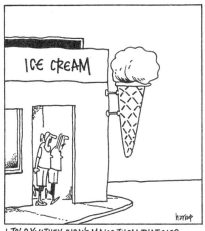

I TOLD YOU THEY DIDN'T MAKE THEM THAT SIZE...

Ready ... set ... go!

Have you compared your portions with those listed in How Much Is Enough —But Not Too Much? (page 32). If not, schedule 15 minutes to do so—mark it on your day planner! Most people are confused about serving sizes. Restaurant portions aren't a good guide!

Check your day planner's **Eating icon** each day you eat amounts that are just "enough," according to the guidelines you've learned.

Notes to Myself

I can picture myself eating well in moderate amounts. I'm going to record the foods I overeat and gradually adjust the quantity:

Time of Day	Foods I Eat "Too Much"	Amount I Eat Now	Amount That's "Enough"

Dine-o-Mite:	Don't be fooled: Salads doused with dressing can be calorie heavyweights. Ask for dressing on the side.	🍐	👟	♡
Today:				**1**
Soul Provider:	Healthy bodies come in a wide range of shapes, sizes, and weights. You can be successful, happy, and positive at any size.	🍐	👟	♡
Today:				**2**
Go with the Flow:	Can we talk? The color of your urine signals your hydration level. Dark gold means you need to drink more fluids. Pale yellow or no color indicates sufficient intake.	🍐	👟	♡
Today:				**3**
Stats Quo:	The U.S. produces 3,700 calories per capita daily. Most women require half that amount, most men about two-thirds.	🍐	👟	♡
Today:				**4**
Heavy Breathing:	By positioning your body and protecting your back from strain, strength-training machines are often safer than free weights.	🍐	👟	♡
Today:				**5**
Rites of Spring:	Take exercise off your "To Do" list and do what the sports ads suggest—just *do* it! Make active living a priority.	🍐	👟	♡
Today:				**6**
Moving Moment:	Seven days without exercise makes one weak. You'll lose 10 percent of your flexibility, muscle strength, and endurance with each decade —unless you exercise.	🍐	👟	♡
Today:				**7**

Beauty and the Best: When we were young, we tooted kazoos, played hopscotch, and danced in the dark. Why not now? Life is meant to be lived!

Make Your Calories Count

Make your calories count without counting calories. The smartest food choices provide the *most* food value for the *least* number of calories— plenty of nutrients for health and vitality, and fewer calories from fat and sugar to add unwanted pounds.

Healthy foods can be the least expensive in the supermarket, especially when they have minimal processing and packaging. Your smartest food choices include:

- Grain Products such as whole-grain bread, cereals and pasta, and brown rice; fresh and frozen Vegetables and Fruit. These choices are packed with vitamins, minerals, trace nutrients, and fiber.
- Low-fat, low-sugar Milk and Alternatives such as yogurt, tofu made with calcium, or dark green vegetables. Plant-based Milk Alternatives are included in this group for their calcium content.
- Meat and Alternatives that are low in fat, including lean fish, lean meat,

and skinless poultry. Plant-based Alternatives such as beans and lentils are a source of fiber. All are good sources of iron and protein. The *Never Say Diet!* Food Circle, found on page 126, can help you with your choices.

Skimming the Fat

The *Never Say Diet!* Food Circle shows food as a continuum from most nutritious to least nutritious. No single food is all good or all bad.

- Inner Circle foods are nutrient-dense and a calorie bargain. Choose them often.
- Outer Circle foods are somewhat nutritious. You have to consume more calories to get the same amount of nutrients found in Inner Circle foods. Choose them in moderation.
- Other foods are least nutritious. Most are high in fat and sugar, but low in nutrients. Use occasionally and in small quantities.

Notes to Myself

With the *Never Say Diet!* Food Circle as a guide, I'll list everything I eat or drink today, under the following headings. I'm on track if most of my foods are from the Inner Circle and few are Other Foods.

Inner Circle	Outer Circle	Low-Cal Others	High-Cal Others

Stats Quo:	Studies show that people considered least fit have death rates three to five times higher than those considered moderately fit. Get a move on!	🍐	👟	🤍
Today:				**8**

Goal Getter:	"Lite" can mean "light-colored" or "light" in taste. Compare the total fat content of any "lite" food against the regular version: The label tells the story.	🍐	👟	🤍
Today:				**9**

Binge Buster:	Physical exercise helps blunt the craving for high-fat foods. The very best way to lower your fat intake? Eat a variety of foods from the major food groups.	🍐	👟	🤍
Today:				**10**

Poultry in Motion:	Vertical roasting drains away fat. Ask any cooking store for a stand-up chicken roaster.	🍐	👟	🤍
Today:				**11**

Just Desserts:	Moderate indulgences help you relax. The occasional cookie, slice of cake, or chocolate bar won't hurt—as long as you don't overdo it.	🍐	👟	🤍
Today:				**12**

Soul Provider:	Look at your world through new eyes. Notice the color of leaves, the arch of a flower, the trill of a baby's laugh.	🍐	👟	🤍
Today:				**13**

Herb 'n' Renewal:	Make meals zestier—literally! Grate in a little orange, lime, or lemon zest, or sprinkle on some juice. No need for salt!	🍐	👟	🤍
Today:				**14**

Beauty and the Best: Visualize yourself in motion. Now move your body for one minute, and pay attention to how you feel. You're on your way!

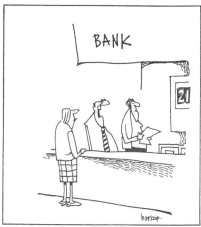

WILL YOU GET MRS. ATKINSON'S TWINKIES FROM THE SAFETY DEPOSIT BOX...?

The Choice Is Yours

Start with changes that are easy and appealing. Plan healthy substitutions, making only one or two changes at a time. Allow yourself time to adjust to your new choices.

Count Yourself In

Eat more and gain less! Upgrade your choices. Referring to the *Never Say Diet! Food Circle* on page 126, replace some of your Other foods with Outer Circle foods, and some of your Outer Circle choices with Inner Circle foods.

Imagine giving your body only foods of the highest quality! Think how energetic your body will *feel!* You'll feel satisfied longer, too.

Ready ... set ... go!

Make a plan—then follow it! Easier said than done? What might interfere with your plan to upgrade food choices? Think about how you could overcome obstacles.

Check your day planner's **Eating icon** each day you replace some of your usual choices with new improved ones.

Notes to Myself

I visualize myself giving my body only the most nutritious foods. I'll upgrade my choices, one at a time:

Time of Day	Usual Choice	New Improved Choice	Amount

Soul Provider:	You've given all day—now take! Take a walk. Take a bubble bath. Take a break. Tune in to your body rhythms. Savor the moment. Discover the joy.			**15**
Today:				
Leaps and Bounds:	Keep a pair of socks and exercise shoes in your desk drawer, briefcase, or in the trunk of your car. Planning ahead means planning for success.			**16**
Today:				
Goal Getter:	Aerobic exercise needs oxygen to fuel the muscles: Oxygen helps burn fat. That's why aerobic activities slim and trim.			**17**
Today:				
Stats Quo:	A daily average of 4,000 milligrams of sodium (the equivalent of two teaspoons of salt) erodes our skeletons by two percent a year.			**18**
Today:				
Binge Buster:	Serving for serving, juice offers more calories and less fiber than fresh fruit, with only minor appetite reduction.			**19**
Today:				
Nothing to Lose:	Is too much work and too little sleep derailing your good intentions? Return to your 3 E's: Each day is a new beginning.			**20**
Today:				
Moving Moment:	By lifting your mood, increasing blood flow, and toning your body, exercise gives your sex life a boost, too. What a turn-on!			**21**
Today:				

Beauty and the Best: Ours is a world of wonders: the deserts, the forests, the oceans, the frozen regions north and south. Life pulses all around us, with a comforting, steady beat.

39

Practice Power Snacking

Power snacking is one of life's many little pleasures. Conscious and purposeful, it satisfies your cravings and gives you the energy to be active until your next meal. Unlike uncontrolled, absent-minded snacking, power snacking has no legacy of guilt and regret.

Power snacking works *with* your body. Unconscious snacking works *against* it. You need to do a little planning ahead to power snack, keeping delicious, healthful treats on hand so you have them when you want them. If you're worried about temptation, stock small quantities.

Choose something you'll enjoy— that's what makes snacking pleasurable. Go for quality—something that makes you feel good even after you've eaten it. Sit down and give yourself time to eat slowly, so you can savor and appreciate the food. Give your body a chance to notice, and stop when you're satisfied.

Plan to Succeed

Decide for yourself what you want to eat, but make it easy by having on hand the foods and drinks you need. We suggest you carry a little notepad to make shopping lists. Consider checking one or two grocery store flyers during a coffee break once a week. Stocking up on specials can make it easier to stick to your plans as long as ample supplies don't tempt you to overeat.

Observe your snack pattern for four days without making any changes. If you answered "Yes" or "Usually" to each of the questions in the Notes to Myself section below, your power-snacking potential is excellent. Most people answer "No" or "Sometimes" to some of these questions. That's normal.

Notes to Myself

I love to snack! How's my power snacking potential?

	Yes	Usually	Sometimes	No
I limit snacking to a specific time-frame— say, 15 minutes—midway between meals.				
I limit snacks to a moderate amount—e.g., one medium muffin or a serving of yogurt.				
My snack choices are from food groups— e.g., an apple instead of apple pie.				
I can resist eating cues that aren't hunger-related—e.g., TV ads, fatigue, anger, or boredom.				

Goal Getter: Program yourself for success. Fuel your exercise with a low-fat meal three to four hours before working out, and a light snack one hour before.

22

Today:

Moving Moment: Exercise builds muscle—nature's fat-consuming engine. As you get stronger, your body gets better at burning calories.

23

Today:

Binge Buster: Meatless can be marvelous: Try bean burritos, pasta primavera, or veggies stir-fried in broth with a side serving of brown rice. Or wrap sauteed veggies in a tortilla.

24

Today:

Soul Provider: Permanently changing your weight also means changing your life: finding new interests, skills, pleasures, and dreams, and seeking new solutions to old problems.

25

Today:

Discomfort Zone: Stretching and strengthening exercises reduce the risk of injury by lengthening muscle-connective tissue and lubricating the joints.

26

Today:

Stats Quo: If only one adult in ten began a regular walking program, the U.S. medical system could realize annual savings of $5.6 billion in heart-care costs.

27

Today:

Sylph Esteem: Stand naked before the mirror. Your body is yours alone. Respect yourself at any size, at any weight.

28

Today:

Beauty and the Best: Take time—make time!—to relax each day. Soak in the tub, read a book, go for a walk, meditate and reflect. This is your time for you.

Put Yourself in the Picture

Plan a specific snack for the time of day you're most likely to overeat. If you tend to eat or drink continuously, select a definite time and duration to snack. Sip water during the rest of the time you'd otherwise be nibbling. This may be hard at first, but it does get easier!

Choose a snack that's familiar, pleasing, and convenient. Make it one serving, from one or two food groups. (A tip: High-fiber carbohydrates "stick to your ribs" and satisfy cravings.) Have some water or plain tea with your snack. If you prefer coffee or a diet drink, limit it to one serving.

Allow enough time to break from other activities, sit down, and focus on the snack. Plan a variety of snacks for different times so you won't get bored. You won't always choose a healthy snack—we're all human! But make sure you think about your choice first. Choose the healthier snack next time!

Ready ... set ... go!
When will you start your plan? Make sure it happens by setting a date. Is there anything that might interfere? If so, how will you overcome any obstacles?

Check your day planner's **Eating icon** each day you practice power snacking.

Notes to Myself

I visualize myself snacking well and with awareness. How does it *feel* to be the person in that picture?

Goal Getter:	"Brain food" is probably an old husband's tale. Stimulate your brain the tried-and-true way: Read a book, share interesting conversation, or do a crossword puzzle.	🍐	👟	♡
			29	
Today:				
Binge Buster:	Extra fat lurks in battered, fried, and creamed foods. Go for the straight goods! Perk up the flavors of plain foods with spices and fresh peppers.	🍐	👟	♡
			30	
Today:				

Beauty and the Best: Friends are the flowers in life's garden. Appreciate and nurture them. Let them bask in your sunlight and love.

Comforting Carbs

Hot bread! Pasta! Pastries! They're called "comfort foods" for good reason. They're carbohydrates—foods high in starches or sugars, or both. They're also your body's most efficient source of fuel, quickly converting to energy.

High-carbohydrate foods trigger your brain's release of serotonin—a feel-good chemical that tricks the body into feeling full faster and leaves you relaxed, comfortable, and satisfied after eating. No wonder every culture has its share of deliciously appealing, easily digested "comfort foods." Noodles, breads, pancakes, and rice are popular everywhere—and pizza knows no international boundaries!

Don't Get Caught Napping!

Do you yearn for an after-lunch siesta? You may be able to slough that midday slump if you don't overdo the carbs at your noon meal. Save those pasta entrees for dinner, when a pleasantly drowsy after-effect is more welcome. Balance lunch carbohydrates with low-fat, high-protein foods (lean fish, chicken, meat, beans, lentils) and high-fiber veggies.

To Know Where You're Going, Know Where You're At

While most of us enjoy our comfort foods, some people experience real cravings for carbohydrates. If you often feel desperate for a carbo fix to boost your mood, you may regularly experience lower-than-normal levels of brain serotonin. It's easy to see how this chemical imbalance can lead to unwanted weight gain.

If this describes you, eat regular, moderate amounts of the foods you crave, combining complex carbohydrates with protein—a whole-grain bagel with chicken; a bran muffin with a slice of cheese; cereal with milk; rice with beans. This may keep your carbohydrate cravings in check.

If changing your eating pattern doesn't help, talk to your doctor.

A Natural High

The immediate satisfaction that sugary snacks provide may come from another brain chemical—endorphins. Endorphins are opiate-like substances linked to many pleasurable activities, including the sensation known as "runner's high."

It's believed that women's endorphin levels drop during the premenstrual phase, triggering the onset of PMS, or premenstrual syndrome. Endorphins enter the bloodstream quickly, which is why some women crave sweets at this time of the month.

MAY

Go with the Flow:	Each liter of sweat excreted means the heart works eight beats a minute faster to pump blood to cool the body. Be kind to your heart. Drink water.			1
Today:				
Incredible Edible:	Raw veggies are a satisfying between-meal snack, especially with hummus or low-fat yogurt dips.			2
Today:				
Stats Quo:	Up to 90 percent of women are dissatisfied with their bodies, say some eating-disorder specialists.			3
Today:				
Just Desserts:	When candy is dandy, satisfy your sweet tooth with a few jelly beans, fruit jellies, licorice, or hard candies rather than creamy, chewy, high-fat choices like chocolate, fudge, caramel, or toffee.			4
Today:				
Twist and Pout:	While strength training, breathe out as you exert yourself, lifting or pressing the weight. Grunts and bulging veins signal pressure buildup, which could lead to dizziness, black-out, or broken blood vessels.			5
Today:				
Soul Provider:	Try to view life's changes as opportunities. Survival of the fittest means survival of the most adaptable, not the biggest and strongest.			6
Today:				
Moving Moment:	Pep up with a walk instead of a high-fat, sugary food. The extra mileage may help deflate your spare tire!			7
Today:				

Beauty and the Best: Past failures don't prevent future successes. How can we learn from experience if we never slip up?

45

Carbo-Rater

Carbohydrates are an important source of food energy, providing about half the number of calories as the same amount of fat. Because they're digested easily, they supply "quick" energy. Scientists recommend that we get one-half to two-thirds of our calories from carbohydrates, to keep our fat and protein intake at reasonable levels. But carbohydrates aren't all created equal ...

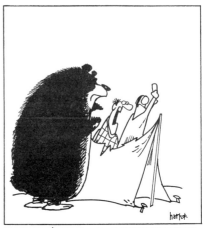

FOR HEAVEN'S SAKE, LOUISE— GIVE HIM THE FUDGIE-WUDGIE CHOCOLATE BAR...!

Complex Carbohydrates

Complex carbohydrate foods are starchy—this group includes whole-grain cereals, bread, pasta and rice, vegetables, dried beans, and lentils. They're minimally processed and nutrient-dense, and are high in vitamins, minerals, and fiber but low in fat. Eating these foods can help keep your appetite in check.

Simple Carbohydrates

Simple carbohydrate foods are high in sugar. Some simple carbohydrates —such as sugar, soft drinks, honey, jams, jellies, syrups, sugary cookies and other baked goods—don't provide many nutrients. They're "empty-calorie" foods. Eating them can actually *increase* your appetite.

Sugar Highs, Sugar Lows

Sugary foods eaten alone are digested and absorbed almost instantly, boosting your blood-sugar levels fast. Easy come, easy go: The energy lift from simple sugars is short-lived. To keep your blood-sugar levels steady, eat regularly and satisfy your sweet tooth with small amounts of simple carbs in combination with their complex cousins or high-protein foods. Enjoy a little jam on whole-wheat bread. Add rolled oats and wheat germ to your cookie recipes. Drink a glass of skim milk with a sweet muffin.

Skimming the Fat:	Tomato, broth, or wine-based sauces are easier on the waistline than gravy or sauces with a cheese or cream base.	🍐	👟	♡
Today:			8	

Waist Not Want Not:	The highest percentage of fat in a woman's diet often comes from mayonnaise, salad dressing, and cheese.	🍐	👟	♡
Today:			9	

Stats Quo:	Canadian snack food retail sales approached the $1 billion mark in 1996, with potato chips sales making up nearly 70 percent of that.	🍐	👟	♡
Today:			10	

Go with the Flow:	A single daily glass of red wine or beer may increase your body's "good" cholesterol. Enjoy —in moderation!	🍐	👟	♡
Today:			11	

Goal Getter:	People who stick with lifestyle changes have three things in common: the belief that they can change, realistic goals, and the ability to accept slips as human.	🍐	👟	♡
Today:			12	

Nothing to Lose:	Get real! Shift your focus from the bathroom scale to health, energy, and vitality.	🍐	👟	♡
Today:			13	

Heavy Breathing:	Keep it lively, keep it fun, keep it movin'! Find an exercise you enjoy, and you'll be more likely to stick with it.	🍐	👟	♡
Today:			14	

Beauty and the Best: Strength becomes a weakness unless you admit your needs. Doing so allows you to be needed, in turn.

Fat City

Fat is essential to health. In our frenzy to eat less, we sometimes forget that. Too little leaves you with sallow skin, dull hair, and a deficiency of vitamins A, D, E, and K. Fat protects us from cold, cushioning our muscles, joints, and vital organs. A little fat goes a long way, but unfortunately, many of us eat too much—much of it in processed foods.

Fat, carbohydrates, and protein provide calories, or food energy. Fat has more than twice the calorie concentration of carbohydrates and protein. That means even small amounts of high-fat foods are packed with calories.

High-fat diets can raise blood cholesterol, increasing the risk of heart attack and stroke. All animals—ourselves included—have cholesterol in their blood. Although pure vegetable oils contain no cholesterol, some oils can cause your body to produce more cholesterol.

The type of fat you eat affects cholesterol levels in your blood, but the amount may be even more important.

Should you worry about how much cholesterol you're eating? Your genetics, your history, your diet, your lifestyle, and whether or not you smoke will determine how your body handles cholesterol.

Fat Facts

Many North Americans derive as much as 40 to 50 percent of their total calorie intake from fat—about 115 pounds (52 kilograms) of fat per person per year. About 50 pounds (23 kilograms) of that is saturated fat (usually from animal sources), which can have negative health consequences.

Straight from the Heart

Healthy hearts depend on healthy lungs. Care for yours: Refrain from smoking, live in a non-industrial area, maintain good posture, and exercise aerobically. If you're a longtime smoker, mastering the 3 E's could make it easier to quit. You may want to make quitting a higher priority than losing weight: smoking a pack a day is as hard on your heart as carrying an extra 80 to 90 pounds (36 to 41 kilograms).

Skim 'n' Trim

- Spread your bread with less or no butter or margarine, or just a little jam.
- Use less or "calorie-reduced" salad dressing.
- Choose low-fat cheeses—let the label be your guide.
- Drink lower-fat milk—skim or 1%.
- Skin poultry before you eat it, and trim all visible fat from meats.
- Limit your intake of high-fat convenience foods and fast foods.
- Bake, roast, broil, poach, or steam instead of frying.
- Substitute unsweetened applesauce for some of the oil or fat in your baking.

Sylph Esteem: *Today:*	Reaching for an unplanned snack? HALT! Are you hungry? Angry? Lonely? Tired? Ask yourself that—and then wait 10 minutes for that snack.	🍐	👟	♡ **15**
Soul Provider: *Today:*	Instead of "doing" all the time, simply let yourself "be." There's no time pressure when you're "being."	🍐	👟	♡ **16**
Incredible Edible: *Today:*	Soft pretzels dipped in a little mustard are a sinfully savory fat-free snack—but take it easy! They aren't calorie-free.	🍐	👟	♡ **17**
Binge Buster: *Today:*	Craving for an extra snack could be your body's signal that you're tired. Getting your Z's can help curb the munchies.	🍐	👟	♡ **18**
Moving Moment: *Today:*	Walking a mile a day means 365 miles a year. If you're of average build, those daily walks will burn 73,000 calories a year!	🍐	👟	♡ **19**
Goal Getter: *Today:*	Use non-stick pans for frying—and skip the oil. Or use spray oils. Reducing the fat in the pan reduces yours, too.	🍐	👟	♡ **20**
Second Helpings: *Today:*	About to reach for that last slice of pizza? Munch some carrot sticks, and save the pizza for tomorrow's lunch.	🍐	👟	♡ **21**

Beauty and the Best: People search for the "meaning of life" as if there were only one. What's the meaning of your life?

Split Personality

Your blood contains two types of cholesterol: HDL (high-density lipoprotein, or "good" cholesterol) and LDL (low-density lipoprotein, or "bad" cholesterol).

- "Good" cholesterol helps zip fat through the bloodstream. It's linked to healthy hearts because it stays on the move until the body excretes it.
- "Bad" cholesterol can stick to the inside of your blood vessels, narrowing the passageway so blood clots can become trapped. That increases the risk of heart disease, circulatory problems, kidney failure, strokes, and other ailments.

Some cholesterol in your blood comes from the food you eat. Your liver makes the rest.

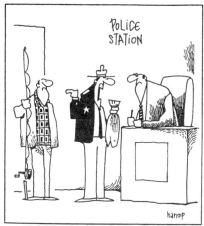

HIS WIFE SAID SHE WANTED POACHED SALMON

Fat 1

Has the fear of fat gotten out of hand? Nutritional scientists say we're becoming too fat-phobic. The best advice? Don't eat too much—of anything.

Fat 2 (Gezundheit!)

Scientists are toiling to create the perfect fat substitute. So far, fake fat has too many flaws. We favor small indulgences of the Real McCoy.

Spread the Word!

Which bread spread do you use? It's not an easy choice.

- Butter is high in saturated fat, which can raise the blood's "bad" cholesterol. Coconut and palm kernel oils also contain saturated fat. (This is why oils that contain no cholesterol can still raise cholesterol in the blood.)
- Margarine is made from unsaturated vegetable oils, which can lower blood cholesterol. But if the oils are hydrogenated or partially hydrogenated, "trans" fat—the unhealthiest of all—is created. If you choose margarine, look for non-hydrogenated products.

But man does not live by spread alone—nor does woman! The big picture's what counts—the quality and quantity of all the fat you eat.

Goal Getter: *Today:*	Diets mean deprivation. Don't cut it out, cut it back—use less mayo or spread, try low-fat milk, or have a bagel instead of a muffin.			22
The Light Stuff: *Today:*	Spreading your daily sandwich with mustard instead of mayo can trim three pounds in a year!			23
A Leg Up: *Today:*	Climbing stairs is great exercise. Daily climbing strengthens your legs and increases your endurance.			24
Binge Buster: *Today:*	Salads aren't a licence to fill. Caesar salad is a high-fat choice. Salads loaded with meat and cheese are loaded with calories, too.			25
Soul Provider: *Today:*	Keep a loose rein on your appetite by watching for signals that tell you when you're hungry and when you're satisfied.			26
Waist Not Want Not: *Today:*	Skim the fat from cooled, homemade stocks and gravies before reheating and serving them.			27
Stats Quo: *Today:*	One guide to body fat estimates that every quarter-inch (0.60 centimeters) you add or lose around the middle equals a pound (0.45 kilograms) of fat.			28

Beauty and the Best: To judge ourselves for being the way we are is like judging the sky for its weather.

Frugal, Fabulous Fiber

High-fiber foods help you manage your weight in several ways. They keep you feeling fuller longer, reducing the temptation to nibble. They carry dietary fats through your system before they're fully absorbed, reducing the amount of fat that gets into your bloodstream. Fiber also slows sugar's entry into the bloodstream, minimizing the highs and lows that make you reach for sugary snacks. Low-fiber diets are linked to appendicitis, heart disease, diabetes, gallbladder disease, and bowel problems. Both soluble and insoluble dietary fiber are important to good health.

High-fiber foods are also often among the least expensive in the store!

Fiber Optics

Fiber is what's left over when your body digests starchy foods. Fiber has no calories. Zip! Zero! Zilch! That's because it passes directly through your gut, from one end to the other.

Of course, the foods that contain fiber have calories, but the higher their fiber content, the fewer calories they contain in each serving.

Most people eat less than half the fiber they actually need, even those who feel they're fiber-conscious. Healthy adults need 20 to 40 grams of fiber each day, but the average intake is about half of that. Eating plenty of fiber-rich foods—such as bran cereal, whole wheat bread, vegetables and fruit, or dried legumes and lentils—will meet your daily fiber needs.

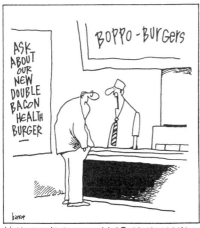

ASK ABOUT OUR NEW DOUBLE BACON HEALTH BURGER

BOPPO - BURGERS

barsot

WE WRAP IT IN A PAGE FROM A FITNESS MAGAZINE.

Beans, Beans, the Musical Fruit ...

We all know the rest of that little ditty: "The more you eat, the more you toot." Some of us know it too well! Fiber doesn't have to become a major—or minor—embarrassment. Increase your intake slowly to avoid feeling gassy and bloated. Drink lots of water, too.

Rinse lentils well before cooking, and soak beans for several hours, cooking them in fresh water. That should mute the musical fruit!

Sylph Esteem: *Today:*	If your crowning glory interferes with active living, consider wash 'n' wear hair. That's the long and the short of it.			**29**
Incredible Edible: *Today:*	Substitute fruit juice for part of the oil in salad dressings and marinades—you'll enjoy full flavor but skimp on the fat.			**30**
Poultry in Motion: *Today:*	Chicken soup really can ease the misery of a cold. It mysteriously breaks up congestion more effectively than other hot liquids.			**31**

Beauty and the Best: Don't get snared in the guilt trap. Occasional, moderate indulgence is a stress-reliever that also strengthens the immune system. Wallowing in guilt can undo the benefits of any relaxing treat.

Sodium: Shakin' All Over

Salt and many other compounds contain sodium, essential for moving water in and out of body cells. We need a daily pinch of salt—but no more! Most of us consume several times that, mainly from processed foods. Too much sodium can upset the body's water balance, leading to bloating and swelling. When you retain fluid, your blood volume increases, raising your blood pressure.

If you have high blood pressure or hypertension, your doctor may advise you to limit your sodium intake. To cut back, season food with herbs instead of salt, read nutrient labels, and choose fewer high-sodium convenience foods and fast foods.

Are You Getting Yours?

Calcium is essential for healthy bones, but many women and men don't meet their daily needs. While bone-building medications and calcium supplements help, so does eating calcium-rich food such as dairy products, dark green vegetables, and tofu made with calcium. Keeping active, particularly with strength-training exercises, is also important. Consume calcium-rich foods at every stage of your life—not just during childhood.

Feel It in Your Bones

High-sodium foods rob calcium from your bones. That means they increase your risk of osteoporosis, a major cause of the frailty, chronic pain, and broken bones that make it hard for many older people to live full, independent lives.

Brittle bones are more than a nuisance: A tight hug, a sneeze, or a cough may be enough to snap a bone in someone with osteoporosis.

Calcium loss affects one in four women, and one in eight men, over 50. Especially at risk are slight, small-boned women with a family history of osteoporosis. Smoking, drinking, and leading a sedentary life all increase the risk, as does a diet high in animal protein.

Blood and Bone

As women enter menopause, the sharp decline in estrogen production causes calcium levels to plummet. The best medicine is preventive: Build strong bones before menopause.

Weight loss can also cause bone loss, so it's probably a good idea to carry a few extra pounds after age 50. While exercise can strengthen bones, over-exercising can weaken them if you lose too much fat and menstruation is interrupted, leading to premature osteoporosis. This has become sadly common in young female athletes.

Go with the Flow: *Today:*	Plain coffee is virtually fat- and calorie-free, but a tall café latté made with whole milk has 180 calories—half of them coming from fat.	🍐	👟	♡ **1**
Goal Getter: *Today:*	Reward yourself with an occasional exercise treat —a new hat, a cozy jacket that wicks away moisture, or a heart-rate monitor.	🍐	👟	♡ **2**
Moving Moment: *Today:*	Consider an active vacation—cycling, rafting, hiking, skiing, swimming—whatever you enjoy the most. Then get out there and do it!	🍐	👟	♡ **3**
Soul Provider: *Today:*	A wise person knows when to seek professional help. If you're down more often than up, talk to your doctor or call your public health department.	🍐	👟	♡ **4**
Binge Buster: *Today:*	A single serving of bran cereal delivers a third of your daily fiber needs. Studies show high-fiber cereal eaters consume fewer calories for lunch.	🍐	👟	♡ **5**
Stats Quo: *Today:*	A new study says we watch TV 40 percent of the time that we don't spend eating, sleeping, working, or doing chores.	🍐	👟	♡ **6**
Incredible Edible: *Today:*	For a low-fat, creamy soup, puree cauliflower in a small amount of its cooking water. Thicken with skim milk powder and season.	🍐	👟	♡ **7**

Beauty and the Best: Reach out to touch another heart; join another soul in this journey we call life.

The Art of Eating: Notes to Myself

Recap time! Jot down everything you eat and drink for one full day. Use "Quick Check" to do a food group tally. Now check to see if your eating is on track.

FOOD/DRINK	AMOUNT
Morning:	
Afternoon:	
Evening:	

QUICK CHECK

Grains ☐ ☐ ☐ ☐ ☐

Veggies & Fruit ☐ ☐ ☐ ☐ ☐

Milk & Alternatives ☐ ☐

Meat & Alternatives ☐ ☐

Water ☐ ☐ ☐ ☐ ☐ ☐ ☐ ☐

Other Foods: Less is Best! ☐

Am I on Track?

☐ Am I eating with awareness, separating eating from other activities, eating in my new eating places, and savoring my food?

☐ Am I spreading my eating fairly evenly over the day, having about half my daily total before I've finished lunch?

☐ Am I eating amounts that are just "enough"?

☐ Am I replacing some of my usual choices with new improved choices?

☐ Am I power snacking?

Binge Buster:	High-fiber cereals and cookies may also be high-fat. Read the labels of all prepared foods, or choose those that are minimally processed.	🍐 👟 ♡
Today:		**8**
Leaps and Bounds:	Don't wait for your exercise shoes to look worn-out before you replace them. Six months of heavy use can sacrifice half their shock-absorbing ability and arch support.	🍐 👟 ♡
Today:		**9**
Dine-o-Mite:	A baked potato in its skin yields fiber with virtually no fat—if you dab on low-fat yogurt instead of a dollop of sour cream.	🍐 👟 ♡
Today:		**10**
Hello to Good Buys:	One small tomato, vine-ripened or not, provides vitamin C, beta-carotene, potassium, B vitamins, and lycopene, a potent antioxidant with many health benefits.	🍐 👟 ♡
Today:		**11**
A Leg Up:	If you're going to walk more than two hours, pack a snack. High-fiber, low-fat crackers, bagels, or fruit are ideal, and low-fat yogurt is refreshing. Take a water bottle, too!	🍐 👟 ♡
Today:		**12**
Just Desserts:	Some frozen yogurts have as many calories as ice cream. Try freezing unsweetened canned fruit and whizzing it in the food processor for a cool treat.	🍐 👟 ♡
Today:		**13**
Goal Getter:	You're more likely to go the distance if you listen to music or books on tape as you move.	🍐 👟 ♡
Today:		**14**

Beauty and the Best: Attitude is a little thing that makes a big difference. If you don't believe in yourself, why should others believe in you?

The Art of Exercise

The Art of Exercise will guide you to:

- Get started
- Write an exercise contract with yourself
- Fine-tune your plan
- Maintain your routine

You're about to discover the joy of movement!

Get with the Program —Enjoy!

What do you want exercise to do for your body? Help you lose weight? Feel more energetic? Strengthen, firm, and tone? Exercise can do all that and more, adding life to your years and years to your life. Really think about your goals and expectations—about what kind of exercise you'd enjoy. Exercise should be fun—if it isn't, you won't want to stick with it.

Before you get started, read the Physical Activity Readiness Questionnaire (PAR-Q) on page 127. It will help you decide if it's safe and healthy to get more active. Talk to your doctor if PAR-Q raises any questions for you.

If you have a disability that limits your activity level, contact a physiotherapist for a custom exercise plan.

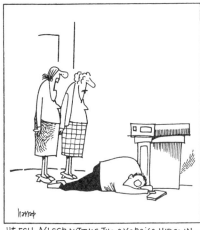

HE FELL ASLEEP PUTTING THE EXERCISE VIDEO IN...

Moving Right Along ...

You know that eating less will slow your metabolism and prompt your body to become efficient at fat storage. You also know that eating too much promotes fat storage. How to achieve a balance? Exercise, the second of the 3 E's, can give your metabolism a boost.

Notes to Myself

I visualize myself as toned, strong, and fit. My blood vessels, capillaries, nerves, muscles, and cells pulse with energy. How does that feel?

Dine-o-Mite: *Today:*	On average, about a third of our food-buying budgets are spent on restaurant food, whether we eat out, take out, or order in.	🍐	👟	♡ 15
Moving Moment: *Today:*	Many concert pianists continue to perform well into their 80s, while most amateur pianists decline in ability. Skills practiced daily stay with you all your life!	🍐	👟	♡ 16
Incredible Edible: *Today:*	Cooked pumpkin, squash, or potatoes mashed with skim milk—but without butter—are excellent low-fat thickeners for homemade "cream" soups.	🍐	👟	♡ 17
Stats Quo: *Today:*	In one year, the average American eats 46 quarts (44 liters) of popcorn and four pounds (1.8 kilograms) of butter. Who wants to be average?	🍐	👟	♡ 18
Waist Not Want Not *Today:*	"Light" beers aren't necessarily lighter in calories than regular beers. Some have about 25 percent fewer calories, because they have fewer carbohydrates.	🍐	👟	♡ 19
Soul Provider: *Today:*	If you can't change a stressful situation, change the way you respond to it. Regular stretching and relaxing can give you a "longer fuse."	🍐	👟	♡ 20
Full Lives: *Today:*	Some people are fit and fat. Others are out of shape regardless of their weight. You can't judge a book by its cover!	🍐	👟	♡ 21

Beauty and the Best: When it comes to your body, you're the expert. A good doctor will ask how you're feeling, then really *listen* to the answer.

Movers and Shakers

Inactivity carries a price—a sluggish metabolism, greater health risks, and less fun in life all 'round. Did someone mention round? You're more likely to add unwanted pounds if you don't move your body. There's nothing wrong with generous proportions if you feel fit and fine. But when extra weight interferes with your enjoyment of life, it may be time for a second look.

Studies show that even moderate physical activity can lead to substantial long-term health benefits, helping prevent heart disease, osteoporosis, diabetes, high blood pressure, and some types of cancer. But the short-term benefits are equally impressive —relaxed muscles, less susceptibility to colds and minor illnesses, more energy for daily activities, and perhaps even a more positive frame of mind.

An optimistic, upbeat outlook on life is healthy. Exercise helps you mentally as well as physically—the ultimate body-and-soul connection! Even mild, regular exercise will help you firm up, making you feel fitter, healthier, and happier. In fact, people who increase their fitness level can lower their cholesterol levels, blood pressure, and risk of heart disease whether their goal is to lose weight or not. It's never too late to begin.

The next few weeks will introduce you to aerobics, strength training, and stretching, showing how all three complement each other. Start slowly and work up gradually. It's not wise to do too much at once. For now, just focus on the joy of simple movement —whatever works for you. Exercising at the right pace means not too slowly or too strenuously. A good test? You should be able to still speak as you exercise.

Make Love, Not Fudge

Too tired to even talk to your partner at night? Exercise relaxes muscle tension—putting a spring in your step and a twinkle in your eye.

Exercise can enhance your love life by improving your stamina, self-esteem, and body image.

Both men and women have greater concentrations of sex hormones in their bodies following a moderate workout. For some, that's a quicker climax.

Notes to Myself

What are my personal reasons to exercise? What kind of exercise would I enjoy? Have I read the PAR-Q on page 127? If not, I'll do it right now!

Moving Moment: *Today:*	The amount of adrenaline you normally produce drops after exercise—one reason exercise is a great de-stressor.			22
Sylph Esteem: *Today:*	A waist is a terrible thing to mind. One size does not fit all.			23
Binge Buster: *Today:*	Mentally divide up your dinner plate. Allow half for vegetables, one quarter or more for grains, and the rest for meat, chicken, fish, or a vegetarian option.			24
Dine-o-Mite: *Today:*	Be a guiltless gourmet. Skip the butter, but not the bun. Ask for milk instead of cream. Ask for vegetables and fruit. Drink water with each glass of wine.			25
Go with the Flow: *Today:*	Steam veggies until they're tender-crisp. Boiling and overcooking leach out precious nutrients.			26
Stats Quo: *Today:*	Recent studies show that about 10 percent of women with lower-than-average weight feel too fat. About 40 percent of average-weight women say the same thing.			27
Skill Power: *Today:*	Foods that proclaim themselves "cholesterol free" may still be loaded with fat. Be a label reader!			28

Beauty and the Best: Feel the wind, sun, rain, and snow against your face; stroke a puppy; touch velvet and straw. Awaken your sensuality!

Aerobics: More Bounce to the Ounce?

So you think aerobics means spandex? Think again—walking, swimming, cycling, and dancing are all aerobic activities. And if you do want to go to the gym, ask about no-bounce classes for deconditioned or size-plus adults. Progressive community centers offer them, and plenty of other fun activities as well.

The object is to work up a light sweat and elevate your heart rate, but leave yourself still able to chat without feeling out of breath.

Building a reputation, fishing for compliments, rising to the occasion, and balancing your checkbook don't count as aerobic exercise! But even simple household tasks—vacuuming, floor-washing, sweeping—do. Choose activities that get you moving steadily over time, delivering plenty of oxygen to your muscles. That's why it's called "aerobic"—because it uses oxygen. What fuels this type of activity? Fat!

How Much and How Often?

Pace yourself! Exercising at a comfortable pace lets your muscles burn more fat while conserving glycogen, a starch stored in the muscles and liver that breaks down to form lactic acid. Exercising too hard increases lactic acid levels in your muscles, producing a stitch in your side or making you stiff and sore.

Stretching before and after aerobic activity also minimizes lactic acid buildup.

Notes to Myself

Am I moving my body enough? Exercising in the range of 11-13 is best.

PERCEIVED EXERTION RATING SCALE																			
1	2	3	4	5	6	7	8	9	10	11	12	13	14	15	16	17	18	19	20

6 = Exercising at an energy level required to get out of bed	7 = Very, very light 11 = Fairly light 13 = Somewhat hard	17 = Very hard 19 = Very, very hard 20 = Total collapse

Moving *Moment:*	Flash! Menopausal women who are physically fit tend to have fewer hot flashes than those who are sedentary.			
Today:				**29**

Stats *Quo:*	Aggressive driving has increased by seven percent every year since 1990. Save your competitive spirit for the tennis court! It's best to arrive home feeling relaxed.			
Today:				**30**

Beauty and the Best: A teacher or an inspiring book can help you see where you are and where you might go from there, but you have to take the journey yourself.

Strength Training: Pecs Appeal

Strength training (also called resistance training) includes any exercise that applies force against gravity. It strengthens muscles, bones, and joints. Imagine having a stronger back for better comfort and posture, sturdier legs for hiking and skiing, denser bones for greater strength and stability. All of these may postpone age-related weakness a decade or longer! Denser bones are more resistant to osteoporosis and fractures, while stronger muscles and joints are less susceptible to injuries.

Strength training also builds muscle, giving your metabolism a boost. That makes you feel peppier—burning more fat, 24 hours a day.

This raises another exercise myth —that you'll look like a football player if you do it. You may get pumped up, but your muscles won't unless you want them to.

How Much and How Often?

Fitness experts suggest strength training for 30 to 45 minutes, two or three times a week. You may want to work your way up to that commitment.

You need balanced muscle development to move your body efficiently and avoid injuries. Walking and jogging strengthen the muscles down the back of your body. You can strengthen the muscles down the front of your body with resistance training.

Which specific exercises are best for you? We recommend that you consult a certified fitness instructor to build your strength-training program. If you want to strengthen and tone muscles without increasing bulk, use smaller weights and gradually increase the number of repetitions, or "reps."

Notes to Myself

I'm eating well, and starting to move my body more. How do I feel about this? How do I feel about me?

Heavy Breathing: *Today:*	Count out loud and you won't forget to breathe during your workout! Holding your breath raises your blood pressure.			**1**
Moving Moment: *Today:*	Tighten your butt and gut muscles each time you wait in a line-up. Let those idle minutes work for you, rather than against you.			**2**
Goal Getter: *Today:*	You won't forget to exercise with an alarm clock on your desk. Hit the pavement or the gym when it rings—no excuses!			**3**
Sylph Esteem: *Today:*	An estimated 20 percent of women on college campuses binge and purge with frequency. How did food become the enemy?			**4**
Go with the Flow: *Today:*	A two percent sweat loss during exercise can result in a 20 percent loss of performance. Boost your energy level! Water is calorie-free!			**5**
Soul Provider: *Today:*	Don't short yourself on sleep. Traffic accidents routinely increase on the first day of Daylight Savings Time, and routinely decrease the day after it ends, when we've slept an extra hour.			**6**
Stats Quo: *Today:*	A recent study showed that 40 percent of the weight dieters lose is lean tissue, while 80 percent of the weight exercisers lose is fat.			**7**

Beauty and the Best: Nature's wheel is always turning. You'd never have a rainbow without a little rain.

Stretching: Freedom to Move

Gentle, controlled stretching will increase your flexibility, helping to prevent injuries, cramping, fatigue, and other problems, such as low back pain. Stretching allows your body to work better and with less effort in a maximum range of motion, making everyday activities easier.

Older people often feel stiff. Gentle stretching and moving keeps you limber longer. Even seniors in nursing homes now do strength training and controlled stretches. The fountain of youth lies within!

Focusing on your breath as you stretch enhances both concentration and relaxation. Stretching is a great way to relax and feel "easy." Do it regularly to create more Ease in your life—the third of our 3 E's for healthy living. We'll talk about Ease a little later. For now, let's step up our thinking about the Art of Exercise!

How Much and How Often?

Stretch three to five times a week, before and after exercise. Hold the stretches a little longer after exercise, when your muscles have warmed up. Hold your warm-up stretch eight to ten seconds. After your walk or workout, stretch each muscle group for 15 to 30 seconds.

Try to be aware of your muscles as you stretch and hold each pose, moving gently without straining, bouncing, or jerking yourself into position. Be sure to exercise both sides of your body. A certified instructor can show you how.

Hush Hour

Taking time to de-stress may mean making time to de-stress. Lie on a flat, hard surface, with one hand on your tummy and the other on your chest. Inhale slowly through the nose, so your stomach contracts. Imagine that your navel is touching your spine. Exhale slowly and deeply through the mouth, so your stomach puffs out. Ahhh!

Notes to Myself

I know about the benefits of exercise—now I'll put it into practice. Is this the fun part? Am I having fun yet? If not, why not? How do I feel?

Binge Buster:	With 90 percent of its calories coming from fat, cream cheese is more like butter or margarine than cheese. Treat it as a spread instead of a sandwich filling.	🍐	👟	♡
Today:			**8**	
Goal Getter:	Your body absorbs most vitamin and mineral pills better if you take them at mealtime. If you're taking two or more tablets of the same type each day, divide the dose between meals.	🍐	👟	♡
Today:			**9**	
Moving Moment:	Studies show that people who exercise regularly are most likely to maintain weight loss. Those who watch a lot of TV are most likely to regain lost weight.	🍐	👟	♡
Today:			**10**	
Stats Quo:	More than 50 percent of heart disease—the leading cause of death in the Western world—is preventable or reversible through positive lifestyle change.	🍐	👟	♡
Today:			**11**	
Go with the Flow:	The average woman needs to consume about three times her body weight in water every seven months. Our bodies are 60 to 70 percent water.	🍐	👟	♡
Today:			**12**	
Soul Provider:	Plan ahead to avoid stress. Shop when it's slow; leave for work a few minutes early; write holiday greeting cards in the fall.	🍐	👟	♡
Today:			**13**	
Incredible Edible:	Shake some dried chili flakes over whole-grain pasta for a zippy, zesty taste. Penne from heaven!	🍐	👟	♡
Today:			**14**	

Beauty and the Best: Where do you want to be in a week, a month, a year? How do you plan to get there? Write down your goals and check them from time to time. Are they the right goals for you?

Get Started

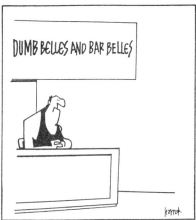

DUMB BELLES AND BAR BELLES

HOWARD BEGAN TO SUSPECT THAT HE MIGHT HAVE
CHOSEN A BETTER NAME FOR HIS WOMEN-ONLY GYM.

If you haven't already started moving your body, this step is a must! For now, don't measure your goal in inches or pounds. Don't measure it by marathons or mountains, either. Just move your body in a way that feels good, and repeat that experience over and over again.

Begin with the 3 E-sy Basics (page 6), gradually advancing to one short daily walk. Keep moving for at least 10 minutes. Exercise at least every second day, but keep active every day! That's all there is to it! If you're already exercising regularly, you'll soon progress to the second step.

Last week, you asked yourself if you were having fun. It wasn't a frivolous question. Exercise that isn't fun isn't exercise you'll stick with.

Notes to Myself

I'll track my activities this week. If there are times I could exercise, but don't, I'll think about why I don't.

THIS WEEK'S EXERCISE RECORD					
Day of Week	Time of Day	Duration	Exercise Opportunity	Took It? Yes? No?	Reason?
Monday					
Tuesday					
Wednesday					
Thursday					
Friday					
Saturday					
Sunday					

Garden of Eatin': *Today:*	A baked potato loses 60 percent of its vitamin C content if left to stand for an hour after cooking. Get 'em while they're hot!		🍐	👟	♡ 15
Waist Not Want Not: *Today:*	Travel light! Carry your own fresh veggie snacks to supplement or replace high-fat, low-fiber air fare.		🍐	👟	♡ 16
Leaps and Bounds: *Today:*	Since you take in more air when you exercise, you also inhale more pollutants. Avoid exercising near heavy traffic. And stay indoors when the air gets too hazy.		🍐	👟	♡ 17
Hello to Good Buys: *Today:*	A recent study showed that potatoes offer the greatest satisfaction after eating. They're up to seven times more filling than an equal-calorie portion of croissants.		🍐	👟	♡ 18
Stats Quo: *Today:*	In a survey of 8,000 women who exercised regularly, 40 percent said a light workout made them more easily sexually aroused. Nearly a third wanted sex more often.		🍐	👟	♡ 19
Soul Provider: *Today:*	Get out of your head and into your heart. Getting older means getting better.		🍐	👟	♡ 20
Incredible Edible: *Today:*	If you knew sushi like we know sushi... Some fish oils guard against high blood pressure, diabetes, cancer, arthritis, and even allergies.		🍐	👟	♡ 21

Beauty and the Best: No body's perfect, so why should yours be?

Put Yourself in the Picture

- Are you living more actively and finding ways to move during the day?
- Are you paying more attention to how your body feels when it's in motion?
- Are you exercising aerobically—walking, dancing, running, cycling—for at least 10 continuous minutes at a time?
- Are you exercising at least every second day?

If you can check each question "Yes," you've made a great start! Use the chart below to write a new exercise plan. Start it tomorrow.

Ready ... set ... glow!

Check your day planner's **Exercise icon** each day you carry out your plan.

Reward Time!

Exercise may be its own reward, but you deserve to treat yourself! Consider buying yourself a pedometer, a Walkman, or a great new T-shirt to keep you going.

Truce or Consequence

If you're getting out of breath, your body's saying "Slow down!" Any discomfort should be mild and brief. "No pain, no gain" is a myth. Call your doctor at once if you experience chest pain. And don't ignore persistent pains in your feet, knees, or anywhere else!

Notes to Myself

EXERCISE PLAN					
Day of Week	Time of Day	Duration	Activity/ Exercise	Obstacles	Solutions
Monday					
Tuesday					
Wednesday					
Thursday					
Friday					
Saturday					
Sunday					

Stats Quo: *Today:*	North American adults weigh an average of eight pounds (3.6 kilograms) more than they did a decade ago.	🍐	👟	♡ 22
Go with the Flow: *Today:*	Don't wait until you feel thirsty to drink. By the time you're aware of your thirst, you're already dehydrated.	🍐	👟	♡ 23
Heavy Breathing: *Today:*	Exercise promotes higher energy levels, fewer stress-related ailments, a toned body, and an improved sex life.	🍐	👟	♡ 24
Poultry in Motion: *Today:*	Prebasted turkeys are injected with saturated fats. No added fat is needed! Cover the bird during the first half of the roasting period, and it will stay juicy without basting.	🍐	👟	♡ 25
Just Desserts: *Today:*	Eating one cookie rather than three means one-third the calories with all the taste. Eat slowly and enjoy the cookie more.	🍐	👟	♡ 26
Soul Provider: *Today:*	Plan the great escape: Lose yourself in a movie, a novel, a country drive, or a stirring piece of music. Making time for yourself is a healthy habit to cultivate.	🍐	👟	♡ 27
Nothing to Lose: *Today:*	Focus on how you *feel*—not on how others think you should *look*.	🍐	👟	♡ 28

Beauty and the Best: Live in the moment. Yesterday is a memory; tomorrow, a hope and a promise. Today is the day that counts.

Setting Goals: How Do I Get There from Here?

Achievers tend to be goal-setters. They decide where they want to go, and then decide how they're going to get there. Setting one huge goal—I'm going to run the marathon!—is both daunting and discouraging, because the goal is so far in the future. But setting many smaller goals—I'm going to start a walking program, and gradually work up to jogging—sets your goals in the present and makes them more achievable. Your motivation levels soar because you can expect a regular reward of positive self-talk—hey, way to go!—each time you meet your target.

Smart goal-setting has three important qualities: Your goal should be be realistic, attainable, and specific. Not "I'll be a runner someday," but "I'll start training 10 minutes a day this week, and work up to 15 minutes next week."

Pop Quiz

Quick! Name three key parts of a balanced exercise program. You get full marks if your list includes:

- Aerobics
- Strength training
- Stretching

Look for all three in a fitness class.

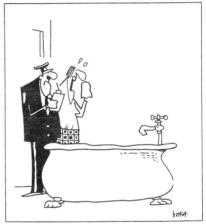

I TOLD HIM TO GO WITH THE FLOW AND HE SLIPPED DOWN THE DRAIN...

Notes to Myself

I'll set some exercise goals, and do some thinking about how and when I'm going to reach them. How does that make me feel?

Skill *Power:* *Today:*	Use this test to slow down your eating and control your portions: Try eating with a blind-fold, stopping as soon as you're satisfied.			29
Go with *the Flow:* *Today:*	Every couple of pounds (one kilogram) of weight lost during exercise is the equivalent of four cups (one liter) of fluid. The more you exercise, the more you need to drink.			30
Heavy *Breathing:* *Today:*	Perk up your walking with intermittent bursts of jogging or speed-walking. Both are metabolism-boosters.			31

Beauty and the Best: Life flows smoother when you aren't too quick to grab what you want and reject what you don't.

Write Your Own Contract

Design Your Plan

Getting FIT takes three things:

- **Frequency**: Exercise regularly. Every second day is better than three days on, four days off. Rest is important, too—take one or two days off during the week, but not two days in a row.
- **Intensity**: Strive for a steady pace that has you breathing hard but still able to carry on a conversation. When you're breathless, your muscles aren't getting enough oxygen to burn fat effectively.
- **Time**: Start with a warm-up period of five to ten minutes to gradually increase your heart rate and warm your muscles. Move on to the brisker aerobic phase, keeping it up for 20 to 30 minutes. If you like, add 10 minutes of strength training, since your muscles are already warm. End with a cool-down period, moving at a slower pace for five to ten minutes for gentle recovery. Total: 30 to 60 minutes.

Put Yourself in the Picture

Starting any exercise program is the hardest step. Sticking with it is the next-hardest! Keep your goals flexible so they'll continue to work for you. Only you can tailor your exercise program to your life. The best way to do that is to write a contract with yourself for the type of physical activity you enjoy.

If you're following the FIT principle, you're ready to write your contract. Take a few moments to again review PAR-Q, page 127.

Check your day planner's **Exercise icon** each day you follow your contract.

Notes to Myself

I visualize myself exercising regularly, anticipating and sidestepping possible obstacles, and making it happen!

EXERCISE CONTRACT				
Frequency:	_____ times per week			
Intensity:	Brisk, but able to carry on a conversation or _____ to _____ on the Perceived Exertion Rating Scale, page 62			
Time:	Warm up _____ minutes		Aerobic _____ minutes	
	Strength _____ minutes		Cool down _____ minutes	
Total:	_____ minutes			

Incredible Edible: *Today:*	Make a vegetarian variation of luscious lasagna with part-skim ricotta cheese and part-skim mozzarella, omitting the meat from the tomato sauce.		**1**
Heavy Breathing: *Today:*	Inhale through your nose and exhale through your mouth as you strength-train. Forgetting to breathe increases abdominal pressure, risking a hernia and a permanent pot belly.		**2**
Just Desserts: *Today:*	You could eat 12 cups of plain popcorn before consuming as many calories as you'll find in a single piece of apple pie.		**3**
Stats Quo: *Today:*	Americans shell out an average of $35 billion a year for weight-loss products.		**4**
Go with the Flow: *Today:*	Don't overlook the importance of water when you travel by jet. General rule of thumb: Drink an eight-ounce (250 milliliters) glass every hour you're airborne.		**5**
Moving Moment: *Today:*	HDL or "good" cholesterol isn't something you'll find on a label: Your body makes it. To boost "good" cholesterol levels, exercise more and quit smoking.		**6**
Goal Getter: *Today:*	Let go of guilt about yo-yo dieting and weight cycling. Studies show that past gains and losses needn't hinder today's healthier habits.		**7**

Beauty and the Best: You are a miracle of nature. Love your body. Love yourself. You're part of this beautiful world.

Obstacles, of Course!

So now you've set achievable goals, and started exercising regularly, right? We hope so—but life's not always like that. It starts to rain, you've got to grocery shop, your youngster needs help with his homework. Remember what you learned about Inner Wisdom and Outer Distractions? They don't just apply to Eating! You can work around Outer Distractions: The gym has no rain, dogs, or stop lights! I'll shop at a different time! I'll exercise when school's in session or ask someone else to tutor!

Connecting with your Inner Wisdom takes more work. A little positive self-talk always helps.

- "I just can't get started." I'll set a smaller goal. If necessary, I'll refocus on the 3 E-sy Basics (page 6).
- "I don't have time." I know everyone has an equal number of hours in each day, so I'll prioritize. I'll also take three 10-minute activity breaks instead of one half-hour session. And I'll do some doubling-up—doing sit-ups in front of the TV, or walking on the treadmill while I'm reading.
- "Exercise is boring." Not with activities I enjoy. Maybe this is the time to enroll in a ballroom dancing class. Or to finally learn how to swim.
- "I'm too tired." It's important to listen to my body! I'll take it slow, and gradually work up. I know exercise is energizing, and will also help me sleep better tonight.
- "It takes too long to see results." A more positive frame of mind, more spring in my step, and more oxygen going to my cells sound

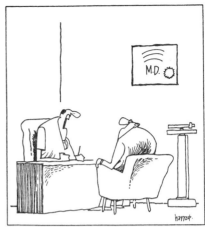

I ADVISE SIX TO EIGHT GLASSES OF WATER A DAY OR FIVE MINUTES IN THE SHOWER WITH YOUR MOUTH OPEN.

pretty immediate to me. I'll remind myself of what this lifestyle planner asked me in January: How would I feel today if I'd been eating well, exercising regularly, and relaxing daily during the past six months? How do I feel today?

- "I'm too out-of-shape to try." Everyone benefits from exercise, whether they want to shed pounds or not. I'll join a no-bounce, size-plus fitness class. I know that how hard I exercise counts a whole lot less than how often. I'm going to have some fun!

H_2O on the Go

Try this easy hot-weather sports drink to replace electrolytes lost as you exercise. Prepare your favorite sugared, bulk-drink crystals at half-strength, adding a pinch of table salt and a pinch of potassium chloride to the pitcher. Drink after exercising. During exercise, drink plain water.

Heavy Breathing:	Regular exercise helps lower blood pressure, control cholesterol levels, promote weight loss, and improve your mood.			**8**
Today:				
Goal Getter:	Treating yourself to fitness togs will help you view yourself as an "exerciser." Focus on comfort and ease of movement.			**9**
Today:				
A Leg Up:	Pool your resources! Swimming improves muscle tone, and trims inches.			**10**
Today:				
Stats Quo:	It takes 14 minutes—from peeling to packaging—to make one potato chip, but just a few seconds to eat it.			**11**
Today:				
Soul Provider:	To live simply in a complex world, give yourself permission to be flexible and spontaneous, and let the spirit lead. Life is full of surprises!			**12**
Today:				
Binge Buster:	When temperatures soar, cut back on proteins and fats. They increase the body's heat production. Fruits and vegetables are more cooling. Drink plenty of plain water, too.			**13**
Today:				
Leaps and Bounds:	Chill out! Because their sweat glands and basal metabolic rates are more efficient, exercisers stay cooler in summer and warmer in winter than sedentary folk.			**14**
Today:				

Beauty and the Best: You are the sum of the choices you make. Choose to be free in your mind. Choose to be positive rather than negative.

77

Fine-Tune Your Plan

Design Your Plan

If your exercise choice isn't working, find out why. You may have to try several things before you find something you enjoy. Be open to it. Be flexible.

Fine-tuning is a skill you'll use over and over again. Seasons change. So do schedules and priorities. Maybe you're getting fitter, and want to pick up the pace. Increase Frequency and Time before focusing on Intensity.

Maybe you're getting bored and want to try something new. Go for it! Perhaps you'd like to try strength training, or enhance this part of your routine. Don't forget to include gentle, controlled stretching in the warm-up and cool-down phases of your balanced exercise program.

Put Yourself in the Picture

How can you make your exercise routine more satisfying? Should you be getting up a little earlier, finding an exercise buddy, or buying a more comfortable pair of shoes?

If you're trying to lose weight, don't be discouraged by occasional "plateaus"—when weight loss seems to stop. They're normal!

Do you foresee any obstacles to starting your new plan? If so, how will you overcome them?

Check your day planner's **Exercise icon** each day you follow your Exercise Contract—Fine-Tuned.

Notes to Myself

This is a plan that works for me, meeting my needs and my schedule.

EXERCISE CONTRACT—FINE-TUNED		
Fat Burning: Frequency: _____ times per week		
Intensity: Brisk, but able to carry on a conversation, or _____ to _____ on the Perceived Exertion Rating Scale (page 62)		
Time: Warm up _____ minutes	Aerobic _____ minutes	
Cool down _____ minutes	Total _____ minutes	
Strength Training: Frequency: _____ times per week		
Time: _____ minutes		
Stretching: Frequency: _____ times per week		
Time: _____ minutes		

Skinny Dipping:	View a buffet table as you would a restaurant menu. You wouldn't order everything on a menu, so why eat everything at a buffet? Eat smart by sampling just a few dishes.			15
Today:				

Stats Quo:	Three daily cups of coffee, with cream and two spoons of sugar, means a potential 40-pound (18-kilogram) weight gain in a year!			16
Today:				

Heavy Breathing:	Studies show that morning exercisers stick with their programs much more than afternoon and evening ones.			17
Today:				

Moving Moment:	A variety of exercise is as healthy as a variety of food. Varied exercise stretches both mind and body, staving off boredom.			18
Today:				

Incredible Edible:	Genetic research and engineering has given carrots twice as much beta-carotene, a valued antioxidant, as they had in 1950.			19
Today:				

Soul Provider:	Work with your body, breath, and mind. Move more. Eat well. Breathe deeply and relax. You are one with the universe.			20
Today:				

Hello to Good Buys:	Broccoli stalks are loaded with fiber. Even the woodiest parts can be used to make stock for soups and stews.			21
Today:				

Beauty and the Best: Taste the nectar of a fresh, juicy orange; enjoy the crunch of an apple; savor the flavor of homemade soup; eat a chocolate, nibble by nibble. Make the goodness last! Your body deserves the best—good things in moderation.

Attitude Is Everything!

Winners know they're winners—because they tell themselves so! Positive affirmations are an important part of life. They motivate. They stimulate. They're a natural high.

By doing the best for your body, you're becoming the best you can be. Write down your affirmations. Put them in the present tense, rather than in the future. You are the best you can be, at this moment, on this day!

Read your affirmations daily; keep a copy of them in your pocket. When you think of yourself as healthier, stronger, and more toned today, as though you have already realized your goal, you *become* that person you envision.

It can be self-defeating to say "I'm going to lose/gain a pound this week," because weight change isn't always predictable. Telling yourself you'll walk every day at a specific time is a much more attainable goal, with relaxation and fun as immediate pay-offs. If your weight changes in the process, that's a bonus!

What You See Is What You Get

Unharness the power of your imagination! It can take you anywhere at lightning speed—to wooded trails, to the ski slopes, to the pool. Let your imagination soar several times a day. Close your eyes and see yourself meeting your goals—you're a winner, too!

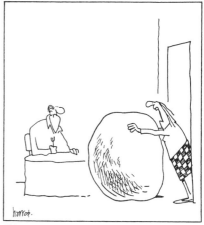

I'M ALLOWED TWO MEATBALLS WITH MY SPAGHETTI.

Notes to Myself

My visualizations and affirmations are deeply personal. I can be anyone and do anything in the theater of my mind. For instance:

Goal Getter:	Pack your gym bag in advance and keep it by the door. The time you save will make it less likely you'll procrastinate, or change your mind about exercising.		🍐	👟	♡
Today:		22			
Incredible Edible:	Mix 'n' match creative vegetable combos to fiber up your life. Choose from cauliflower, broccoli, zucchini, carrots, onions, eggplant, tomatoes, and colorful peppers.		🍐	👟	♡
Today:		23			
Hello to Good Buys:	Fresh foods often cost less than processed foods. Shop with the seasons and save!		🍐	👟	♡
Today:		24			
Poultry in Motion:	The chicken always wings twice. Freeze enough wing tips to make flavorful chicken stock.		🍐	👟	♡
Today:		25			
Heavy Breathing:	If your goal is weight loss, combine strength training with aerobics. Studies show that "circuit training" sheds pounds faster than aerobics alone.		🍐	👟	♡
Today:		26			
Soul Provider:	Stress overload leads to moodiness, sleep loss, lack of concentration, a pounding heart, a high pulse rate, and other problems. Take a break—before you break down!		🍐	👟	♡
Today:		27			
Stats Quo:	In one year, the average American consumes 23 quarts (about 22 liters) of ice cream and 16 pounds (7.2 kilograms) of chocolate.		🍐	👟	♡
Today:		28			

Beauty and the Best: There's freedom in recognizing that all of us have imperfections. Focusing on them as major obstacles gives them too much attention.

Maintain Your Routine

Design Your Plan

Ask yourself if your exercise routine is convenient/inconvenient, enjoyable/not so enjoyable. You're on track if you can check most of these statements "Yes!"

- [ ] I keep my plan handy to remind myself to stay active.
- [ ] I reward myself with little treats —of the non-edible variety!
- [ ] I take note of my sense of well-being and sometimes mention it to others.
- [ ] I look for ways to make activity part of my social life.
- [ ] I ask for specific kinds of support and encouragement from those close to me.

If you aren't on track, see the "Notes to Myself" section below.

Put Yourself in the Picture

Consistency is the basis of any habit —healthy or otherwise. Over the past several months, you've gradually been adopting a number of healthy habits. With visualization and goal-setting, you've made them truly yours.

Many people assume the "program" is over when they finally reach their goals. Exercise is not a temporary measure. Your body needs to keep moving as long as you live. That's why it's important to keep exercise fun. To do that, you have to keep motivating yourself. Find a motivator that works for you—everyone's different.

Check your day planner's **Exercise icon** each day you consciously reinforce your routine by getting the support that you need.

Notes to Myself

Planning ahead will help maintain my routine. How can I make it happen?

SUPPORT I'M GETTING NOW		EXTRA SUPPORT I'LL BUILD IN	
From Myself	From Others	From Myself	From Others

Stats Quo:	An estimated 200 Americans eat a hamburger every second of every day.		🍐	👟	♡
Today:					**29**
Hello to Good Buys:	Pre-cut veggies and bagged salads are fast foods without the fat. Minimize nutrient loss: Buy them fresh and eat them soon.		🍐	👟	♡
Today:					**30**
Heavy Breathing:	Don't be modest. Brag about your exercise gains! You may inspire others to join you, and you will also motivate yourself.		🍐	👟	♡
Today:					**31**

Beauty and the Best: Be good to yourself. You have only one body—treat it with care and respect.

Does Class Action Suit You?

You'll progress toward your goals faster and avoid injuries better when you train under a good instructor. You'll also feel more motivated to keep going when you're part of a group. Here's what to look for:

- The instructor is properly trained and certified by a recognized fitness organization.
- You feel comfortable with the instructor and the other partici-pants. There are absolutely no "put-downs."
- Classes start with a gradual warm-up period of at least 10 minutes. This gets your whole body moving at an easy pace. Light stretching may be included.
- The brisker-paced aerobic component lasts at least 20 minutes. Low-impact classes minimize jumping and bouncing, which helps protect your back and joints. This may be followed by 10 or more minutes of strength-training exercises. Weights may or may not be used.
- Classes end with a cool-down period of at least 15 minutes, devoted to stretching and relaxation.
- You're encouraged to move at your own pace rather than keep up with others.
- The class is small enough for the instructor to keep an eye on every-one. Alternately, assistants offer individual attention.

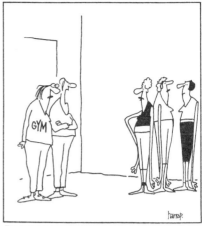

THE INSTRUCTOR TOLD THE CLASS TO STRETCH THEIR LIMBS AND THEN SHE LEFT FOR AN HOUR ...

- The fitness facility has a floor with some spring (exercising on concrete is hard on the legs, feet, and back). It has enough space for you to move around comfortably, safely, and with the level of privacy you prefer.
- The class is held at a time and place convenient for you to attend regularly, preferably two or three times a week. (Supplement those classes with brisk walks on other days.)

I Wanna Get (More!) Physical: Cross-Training

Which exercise is "best"? Whatever turns you on! It's a good idea to try several different types of physical activity so boredom doesn't set in. Varying the pace is called cross-training—you might play tennis one day, hike the next, do a round of "circuit training" at the gym, the next. Whatever you choose, keep moving! It's the secret to success.

Goal Getter:	Looking for food in all the wrong places? Snacks stashed in your briefcase, pockets, car, purse, or night table mean haphazard eating.	🍐 👟 ♡ **1**
Today:		
Sylph Esteem:	The disorder du jour is called "muscle dysmorphia" or "reverse anorexia nervosa." It's the over-exerciser's belief—despite all evidence—that one's body lacks rippling muscles.	🍐 👟 ♡ **2**
Today:		
Binge Buster:	Turn off the tube and adjust the volume on your eating. TV watching promotes mindless eating and snacking, making it easier to forget about the quality and quantity of your food.	🍐 👟 ♡ **3**
Today:		
Soul Provider:	Life is like a swing. It goes up, and goes down—but it always goes up again.	🍐 👟 ♡ **4**
Today:		
Go with the Flow:	You can "chew" water as well as chug-a-lugging it! Water makes up 90 percent of veggies and fruit, 75 percent of meat, and 55 percent of bread.	🍐 👟 ♡ **5**
Today:		
Just Desserts:	Taming the cookie monster is easier if you choose low-fat arrowroot biscuits, ginger snaps, or graham wafers, but close the package after two or three!	🍐 👟 ♡ **6**
Today:		
A Leg Up:	Tell the diet-pushers to take a hike—better still, you take one!	🍐 👟 ♡ **7**
Today:		

Beauty and the Best: Everyone dies. Too few of us really *live.* Make every day count.

The Art of Exercise: Notes to Myself

Check it out! Use this page to make sure you're getting the most out of your exercise routine this week.

Exercise Type:

Frequency:

Intensity:

Time:

How Do I Feel?

Exercise Type:

Frequency:

Intensity:

Time:

How Do I Feel?

Exercise Type:

Frequency:

Intensity:

Time:

How Do I Feel?

QUICK CHECK

Aerobics ☐ ☐ ☐ ☐ ☐ ☐ ☐

Pre-Stretch ☐ ☐ ☐ ☐ ☐ ☐ ☐

Post-Stretch ☐ ☐ ☐ ☐ ☐ ☐ ☐

Strengthening ☐ ☐ ☐

Am I on Track?

☐ Am I keeping physically active every day?

☐ Am I following my daily exercise contract?

☐ Am I reviewing and fine-tuning my exercise contract as circumstances change?

☐ Am I consciously maintaining my routine by getting the support I need?

☐ Am I having fun?

How Can I Have Even More Fun?

Herb 'n' Renewal: *Today:*	Let the contents of an orange, ginger, jasmine, or almond herbal tea bag spice up the cooking water the next time you make rice.	🍐	👟	♡
				8
Goal Getter: *Today:*	Don't give up if you slip up. To falter is not to fail. Review your 3 E-sy Basics—and go easy on yourself!	🍐	👟	♡
				9
Just Desserts: *Today:*	Angel food cake is a smarter nutritional choice than most other cakes because it's low in fat. No egg yolks also means little or no cholesterol.	🍐	👟	♡
				10
Stats Quo: *Today:*	A recent shopping survey found that the more consumers know about nutrition, the less likely they are to believe the health claims on food packages.	🍐	👟	♡
				11
Go with the Flow: *Today:*	We can live several weeks without food, but only a few days without water. Bottoms up!	🍐	👟	♡
				12
Soul Provider: *Today:*	Make a wish on a butterfly as it wings its way to heaven.	🍐	👟	♡
				13
Twist and Pout: *Today:*	Washboard abs? A totally flat stomach is an impossible goal for most people. "Crunches" can strengthen your abdominals, but can't eliminate the fat layer over them.	🍐	👟	♡
				14

Beauty and the Best: Good food is a symphony for the senses—a complex mingling of flavors, aromas, and colors that tempts the palate and satisfies the soul. Focus on each texture and flavor as you eat. Fill the senses as well as the stomach.

The Art of Ease

The Art of Ease will help you discover how to:

- Breathe easy
- Rest easy
- Take it easy
- Speak easy ... and even learn a little ...
- Legal-ease

Pace Maker: Having the Time of Your Life

Life never unfolds as it's "supposed to." It simply happens. Whether you become engulfed in life's tidal waves or simply float on the tide depends on how you respond to the events in your life. The abilities to work with things as they are and accept with grace what you can't change are powerful tools for stress-resistant living. You can rail against life as "unfair," or complain about your "bad luck." In reality, almost all of us face major challenges—if not sooner, then certainly later.

Learning to go with the flow takes practice. You can't usually control things outside your life, but you can control what's within. That doesn't mean keeping a tight leash on your feelings, but rather listening to your body's inner wisdom and the good sense it conveys. It takes quietude and reflection to make the mind–body connection, and confidence to know how to use it. This section will help you learn how.

Moving with Ease

We hope you are eating with newfound awareness and exercising energetically. Now discover the last of the 3 E's! Too many of us define "success" by our wallets instead of our souls. Getting in touch with your inner wisdom means calming the chattering of your mind. It's time to create more Ease in your too-busy life.

Notes to Myself

I can't stress-proof my life, but I can make it more stress-resistant. How do I handle stress each day?

☐ Do I cope without relying on medications, alcohol, or food?

☐ Do I notice stress before a major symptom like a headache or backache develops?

☐ Do I make a conscious effort to release muscle tension often during the day by moving around, stretching, etc.?

☐ Do I express my needs and wants freely to people around me?

☐ Do I get the support and encouragement I need to follow healthy habits?

I'm on track if I answered "Yes" to all or most of these questions. If not, I'm about to boost my EASE quota ...

Moving Moment:	If you often fidget and change position, you may burn enough extra calories to affect your weight. Frequent breaks, in which you move around, also help keep you feeling alert.			**15**
Today:				
Goal Getter:	Match your choice of exercise to your personality. If you're the competitive type, set your sights on a walkathon or fun run to stay motivated. If you enjoy solitude, go for walks or runs on your own.			**16**
Today:				
Go with the Flow:	Filtering coffee helps remove some of the cholesterol-raising compounds naturally present.			**17**
Today:				
Waist Not Want Not:	The numbers on the scale are less important than the notches on your belt. Fat around the middle can carry health risks.			**18**
Today:				
Stats Quo:	Over the course of a lifetime, the average person walks a distance equivalent to twice the circumference of the globe—roughly 310,000 miles or 500,000 kilometers. Go the distance!			**19**
Today:				
Soul Provider:	You can't stop payment on a reality check. Stand by your plan!			**20**
Today:				
Incredible Edible:	Brown rice has more fiber than white. Jazz it up with a little soy sauce, garlic powder, and cayenne pepper.			**21**
Today:				

Beauty and the Best: Some people say that when one door closes, another one opens. We say you have to find the door, and unlock it. Consider the possibilities! Open your heart and your mind!

Stress: Present Tense

Stress affects every system of your body. It gets your heart pumping, stomach churning, adrenaline surging, endorphins soaring. Daily annoyances can add up. The result: an incredible amount of wear and tear on every part of the body, weakening the immune system and leaving you more vulnerable to everything from the common cold to cancer.

Stress can affect your weight. Your body produces more fat-building enzymes during and immediately after stressful situations. For a short time after a stressful event, you may store fat more easily than usual. If stress also leads you to overeat, it's easy to see how living under pressure can add pounds.

Stress can also make some people thinner, especially when emotional upheaval and physical trauma are combined. Extreme physical stress, such as major surgery or a serious burn, boosts a person's need for calories. Anxiety, sadness, fear, and other painful emotions can magnify the effect. Stress can also dull the appetite or speed food through the intestines before it's fully digested. That can mean weight loss.

Making your life more stress-resistant will help every system in your body function better. Creating Ease will also help you find and maintain a stable, healthy weight.

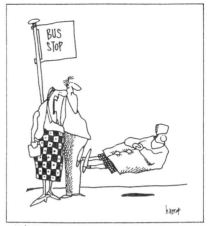

SHE'S ONE OF THE MOST RELAXED PEOPLE I KNOW...

Take Time to Water the Roses

Simplify your life. Get back to your roots. Plant a garden!

The technological age has left many people feeling rootless. Growing some vegetables and a few pretty flowers can literally connect you to the earth. You'll feel you're participating in something basic and worthwhile.

Make your garden small enough that it won't become a chore. If you don't have a little patch of dirt, put a container or two on your patio. Pick up a few bedding plants for instant greenery. But plant a few seeds, too.

Watching your plants grow and thrive will give you a sense of satisfaction unlike any other. Picture yourself adding home-grown tomatoes to a salad, or picking a small bouquet for your desk. Ahhh!

Stats Quo:	Making a list, checking it twice...? Fewer than a quarter of us write a shopping list and stick to it. About a third write a list, but don't follow it.		22
Today:			
Leaps and Bounds:	Too much of a good thing can be bad. Over-exercising can break down muscle tissue, making it harder to lose weight. You'll also risk an injury that could derail your routine for weeks.		23
Today:			
Moving Moment:	Meditate on your muscles. Feel them push, pull, and contract as they work against gravity. You're getting stronger every day!		24
Today:			
Soul Provider:	Life goes on within you and without you. No one is indispensable. Give yourself a break. Relax.		25
Today:			
Incredible Edible:	Take half a dozen pieces of raw veggies or fruit to your workplace each day. Eat them all before quitting time.		26
Today:			
Goal Getter:	You're more likely to snack on fresh vegetables or fruit if they're ready to eat. Prepare them right after buying them.		27
Today:			
Sylph Esteem:	Women who are active tend to have a positive body image and heightened self-esteem.		28
Today:			

Beauty and the Best: Stroking and watching animals lowers stress and blood pressure. Go to the zoo, learn to snorkel, adopt a pet, whistle to a bird. Reconnect with nature to reconnect with yourself.

Ease: Past Tense

We need to relax most when our lives are most stressful. It's hard to stop and smell the roses when you're caught among the thorns, but rather than simply hoping or waiting to relax, you can learn how to relax consciously whenever you want or need to.

We all know people who get "stressed out" more easily than those who take life in stride—even when both face exactly the same annoyance. People who "go with the flow" respond to situations, rather than *reacting* to them as a threat.

Responding, rather than reacting, to your world means paying attention to your body and mind as well as your surroundings. You can become more aware of your body and how it functions—how you breathe, how you move, how you think, and how you sleep. This isn't a selfish thing to do. Others in your life also benefit when you act consciously and purposefully.

Tuning Up

Many people treat their bodies like their cars. They take them for granted until something goes wrong. Even then, they want a quick fix, so they can be back in service without further delay!

Your body is more than a machine. Pay careful attention to it and it will tell you what it needs. Give your body what it needs and it will reward you many times over!

You'll have to be a good listener to "hear" your body's messages. But, hey—you're worth it!

Tuning In

- Treat yourself to a massage on a regular basis!
- Turn down the lights, lie on the floor, and practice your usual stretches as s-l-o-w-l-y as you can—you'll be amazed how that feels!
- Eat a meal blindfolded and really taste each bite.
- Find a quiet, comfortable place and sit—don't lie down—with your eyes closed for one hour.

Stats *Quo:*	Dieting can affect your driving skills. A recent study showed that women who consumed only half the calories needed to maintain their weight had slower-than-normal reaction times.	🍐	👟	♡ 29
Today:				
Go with *the Flow:*	Drink plenty of water—but don't overdo it! We're recommending extra glassfuls, not extra gallons! A "water diet" can land you in the hospital if you flush too many minerals from your body.	🍐	👟	♡ 30
Today:				

Beauty and the Best: Each of us has a special gift to offer the world, whether it is our capacity for love, laughter, understanding, art, or knowledge. Be yourself, and give of yourself.

Breathe Easy

You already have the power to be nutrition-conscious, fit, and energetic. That power is just waiting to be tapped. "Quieting" will enhance your awareness of your body's natural rhythms. It lets you slow down your busy, anxious mind by having you focus on your breath, moment by moment. Quieting is "being" rather than "becoming." Quieting gives you a break from outside distractions—it simply lets you be. We suggest you start with Phase 1, then move on to Phase 2 when you feel ready.

Phase 1

- Sit in a comfortable chair with your back straight but supported, your feet flat on the floor, your knees apart, and your hands resting on your thighs. Or sit cross-legged with a pillow under your buttocks to help keep your back straight. Close your eyes. Begin by noticing your breathing without changing it.
- Start to breathe slowly and deeply, down into your abdomen. If you've been tensing your abdominal muscles, release them.
- As you inhale, think the words "I am." As you exhale, think the word "relaxed."
- Continue to breathe slowly and deeply as you repeat in your mind, "I am ... relaxed."

Do this exercise for several minutes, at least once a day.

Phase 2

- Choose a quiet place where you won't be disturbed for at least 10 minutes. Sit in the balanced position described in Phase 1 and begin breathing slowly and deeply with your eyes closed.
- Focus your attention on each breath as it passes in and out. A good way to keep your attention on your breath is to fold your hands lightly on your tummy. Feel how it rises and falls each time you inhale and exhale.
- Your mind will try hard to interrupt you. When it wanders, release each thought and focus on your breath. Neither dwell on the distractions nor impatiently push them away. Simply notice them, let them go, and return your attention to your breath.

Design Your Plan

What might interfere with your plan to practice Quieting on a daily basis? Address each obstacle, one at a time. If you're uncomfortable with Quieting, use the 3 E-sy Basics (page 6) to get started, gradually staying with it a little longer.

Check your day planner's **Ease icon** each day you spend a few minutes Quieting.

Nothing to Lose: *Today:*	Being very thin is not healthy. It can lower your immunity, putting you at risk for infections. It can also increase your risk of osteoporosis.			1
Stats Quo: *Today:*	Net gains or losses? A recent study showed that 45 percent of nutrition-related Internet Web sites carried advertisements and misinformation.			2
Moving Moment: *Today:*	Hang in there! Psychologists say it takes six to twelve weeks of consistent effort for any new practice to become a habit.			3
Skill Power: *Today:*	Substitute a mug of boiling water for your usual coffee or tea. It's a healthy cup of comfort.			4
In Bod We Trust: *Today:*	Researchers say that of all the smells in the world, the two Americans recognize first are peanut butter and coffee.			5
Soul Provider: *Today:*	Quieting puts us in direct contact with who we are. Think you're too easily distracted? If you can concentrate enough to read a book, you can practice Quieting.			6
Just Desserts: *Today:*	Enjoy such sweet treats as gelatin desserts, skim milk pudding, and fruit crisp. Each contains limited amounts of fat and sugar.			7

Beauty and the Best: Color me serene? Cool tones are soothing. Light blue reduces blood pressure, pulse rate, stress, and body temperature. Green rejuvenates and relaxes. Think flowers, plants, and a sunlit sky—you'll *feel* sunnier, too!

Quieting: Breathing Lessons

Quieting isn't a problem to solve or a goal to be met. You simply become one with your breath—slowly, naturally inhaling and exhaling.

It won't put you into a trance and it won't put you to sleep. By slowing you down, it *will* leave you alert and focused, and at ease in your body and mind. Once you've tried Quieting several times, use this checklist to become aware of its subtle benefits:

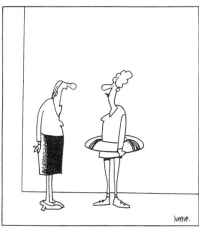

YOU THE ONE WORRIED ABOUT DRINKING EIGHT GLASSES OF WATER A DAY... ?

☐ I notice how busy my mind usually is.

☐ I can sit still a little while longer than I could when I began.

☐ I think about my breathing when I'm forced to wait—it makes me feel more patient when I'm put "on hold."

☐ I feel a little calmer with slow breathing.

☐ I can slow down my eating when I focus on my breathing.

☐ I experience myself as the quiet "watcher" who isn't totally caught up in my daily activities.

Notes to Myself

How do I consciously release tension in my body now? I will stop several times a day, noticing if tension is building in my body. I will tense and release the muscles that need attention. How does this *feel*?

Idle? *Wild!*	Now and then, do absolutely nothing at all. Take a break from exercise. Swing in a hammock. Close your eyes and listen to music. Your "busy-ness" can wait.		8
Today:			
Rate Your Plate:	High-fiber foods keep hunger at bay far longer than foods high in fat. An ample serving satisfies, leaving no urge for seconds.		9
Today:			
Goal Getter:	There are no "bad" foods—only better choices. Hold the fortitude!		10
Today:			
Stats Quo:	By the turn of the century, 40 percent of the paid labor force will work from home. All the more reason to stock the fridge with healthful snacks.		11
Today:			
Moving Moment:	Research shows that people who exercise gain discipline and self-confidence, which enhance all aspects of their lives.		12
Today:			
Garden of Eatin':	For a low-calorie, low-fat salad dressing, combine cider vinegar with salt, pepper, all-vegetable seasoning, a packet of sugar substitute, and a sprinkle of water.		13
Today:			
Full Lives:	It takes more energy to stay as tightly coiled as a bud than to relax and blossom.		14
Today:			

Beauty and the Best: Life is like a candle, keeping the darkness at bay. Sharing the flame enhances its warmth and its glow.

Rest Easy—Progressive Relaxation

Why?

Recognizing tension early will help you respond in healthier ways than developing a headache or sore neck. Curtailing tension and fatigue will make it easier to eat and exercise consciously.

Progressive Relaxation eases muscle tension to make you feel like a limp rag doll. It can also help you get a better night's sleep.

When?

When you're feeling pressured, you probably tense your muscles. Muscle tension is a common sign of stress, and it can easily become a habit. Clenching muscles is tiring. It's one reason you're exhausted at the end of the day, and sometimes have trouble sleeping.

Where?

Choose a quiet, private place. Lie on a mat, carpet, or firm mattress to practice Progressive Relaxation. Close your eyes, breathing deeply and naturally, inhaling energy through your nose, exhaling tension through your mouth. After three deep breaths ...

How?

Focus your attention on one part of your body at a time. Keep breathing while you clench the muscles in that body part for three seconds. Hold, hold, hold ... release. Let that part of your body relax—totally, absolutely, completely. It feels warm, heavy, and relaxed, as though it were suffused with a golden light.

Focus on the next part of your body, section by section, limb by limb. Clench, clench, clench ... release. It also feels heavy and warm. Let it sink deeply into the floor or mattress. It feels very relaxed.

Stick out your tongue as far as you can and scrunch up your face. One ... two ... three ... release. Your face feels very relaxed. You float in a sea of calm, rocked gently by the waves.

Continue to breathe deeply and naturally—in through the nose, out through the mouth. The tension is leaving your body. The tension is floating away.

Inhale energy through the nose; exhale tension through the mouth. Your body feels heavy and warm. The tension is melting away.

Important note: Clench your muscles just enough to feel some tension, and continue to breathe normally as you do so. Hold the tension for just a few seconds. Don't clench your toes if the muscles in your feet cramp easily—instead, put your attention on each foot by gently moving it.

Nothing to Lose: *Today:*	Some obesity has genetic links. We can't choose our parents, but we can embrace a healthy lifestyle.			**15**
Stats Quo: *Today:*	Of 1,000 New Yorkers recently asked to list their favorite foods, more than a third picked pizza. Other faves were hamburgers, ice cream, apple pie, pretzels, and hotdogs.			**16**
Hello to Good Buys: *Today:*	Don't expose yourself to food you want to avoid. Out of sight, out of mind, out of mouth.			**17**
Second Helpings: *Today:*	Boost your veggie consumption by doubling or tripling the amount you'd normally add to soups and stews.			**18**
Go with the Flow: *Today:*	A five to ten percent loss of bodily fluid may produce fatigue, mental confusion, and temperature fluctuations.			**19**
Soul Provider: *Today:*	Your inner beauty and outer grace shine more brightly when you slow down rather than live it up.			**20**
Incredible Edible: *Today:*	If you enjoy an occasional chocolate, don't eat it fast—make it la-a-ast.			**21**

Beauty and the Best: Listen to the music of a waterfall, children at play, pigeons cooing, and different dialects and languages in shops and in the street. Hear the world at work and play, releasing its joyful sound.

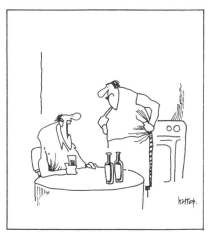

I *DO* DRINK 6 To 8 GLASSES OF WATER A DAY— I JUST PREFER IT WITH ADDITiVES...

Ready ... set ... flow!

When will you try Progressive Relaxation? What might interfere with this plan? How will you overcome obstacles, if any?

Check your day planner's **Ease icon** each day you Rest Easy with some Progressive Relaxation.

Stay Loose!

You can relax tight muscles with gentle self-massage, by taking frequent stretch breaks, by shaking your hands and feet, or by shrugging your shoulders.

Winkin' and Blinkin' and Nod

Progressive Relaxation will help you drift off to dreamland. Mom always called it "beauty sleep"—guess what? She was correct. Sleep loss disturbs several body functions, including the immune system. Losing sleep can make you sick and make you fatter— especially if you snack late at night.

Sleep is essential to good health. Get your share, and luxuriate in it. Other sleep tips:

- Make sure your bedroom is dark at bedtime. Wear a sleep mask if necessary.
- Make sure your bedroom is quiet. Otherwise, wear ear plugs.
- Don't eat, work, or exercise (with certain—ahem!—exceptions!) in your bedroom unless you have no problem falling asleep.
- Keep regular hours, going to bed at more or less the same time every night.
- Create a little bedtime routine—a light snack, a few minutes of Quieting, and Progressive Relaxation.

Soul Provider:	Indulge yourself—or someone else. Let acts of kindness be your legacy.			
Today:				22

Incredible Edible:	An orange contains vitamin C, plus about 150 other substances that may protect your health. A vitamin C pill contains only vitamin C.			
Today:				23

Moving Moment:	A recent study suggests that women who exercise least have twice the risk of colon cancer as women who exercise most.			
Today:				24

Goal Getter:	You can cover a lot of ground by taking small steps, but when you reach a chasm, be prepared to leap!			
Today:				25

Waist Not Want Not:	Prepared popcorn may be labeled "air-popped" but may still contain added vegetable oil or cheese. Read the fine print on the label.			
Today:				26

Rate Your Plate:	Grate raw vegetables and fruit into home-made baked goods, salad, stews, and soups.			
Today:				27

The Light Stuff:	If diet claims seem too good to be true, they are. No one loses five pounds (2.2 kilograms) of fat in a week. Sudden weight loss is mostly a result of lost water.			
Today:				28

Beauty and the Best: Quietude offers many lessons. Heed your inner voice. Listen more than you speak.

Take It Easy

"If you want something done, ask a busy person." We've all heard that old saying. Do people say it about you? It's great to feel valued for making a contribution—but it's stressful to be so over-committed that you feel there aren't enough hours in the day.

It makes you feel guilty when you can't give your "best" because you're overloaded. It's even worse to realize there's no time left for you at the end of a busy day. Making yourself a priority can be difficult, especially if you've never done it before. Learning to say "no" or "maybe next time" is a good start. But learning to ask for the help you need is important, too.

"Busyness" is an addiction. Are you the *only* person who can do these things? Look deep within yourself. Does taking on too much make you feel "needed" or "irreplaceable"? Does finally getting some free time prompt you to volunteer for another chore? Several weeks ago, we talked about having fun. Why not plan for more fun in your life? Why should it all be obligation and work?

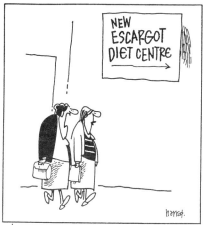

IT'S TAKING ME LONGER AND LONGER TO GET HERE.

Ready ... set ... flow!

- When will you start your plan?
- What might interfere with it?
- How will you overcome obstacles, if any?

Check your day planner's **Ease icon** each day you Take It Easy.

Notes to Myself

How *do* I feel when I take on too much? How *would* I feel right now, if I had time to myself? Am I afraid of "empty" hours? What would I enjoy doing with extra time for me?

Second Helpings:	Drink less coffee but feel just as satisfied— use a smaller cup.			
Today:				29

Binge Buster:	Banana splits for breakfast? Slice a banana lengthwise and top with your favorite cereal, plain yogurt, and chopped nuts. It's a balanced meal in a bowl!			
Today:				30

Heavy Breathing:	Bored with the treadmill? Visualize yourself on an outdoor trail in the woods, by the beach, at the park! Bye-bye, run-of-the-mill routine!			
Today:				31

Beauty and the Best: Think of someone you admire—how she walks, how she talks, how she moves. Imagine yourself as that person, and then practice what you see. Modeling yourself after someone you like and respect is a powerful tool for change.

Design Your Plan

Re-examine your daily commitments. Identify those that you:

- Must do
- Should do
- Can do

Starting with the "Can do's," decide what could be done less often—or dropped altogether. Do the same for the "Should do's" and "Must do's." Don't feel guilty—achievers always prioritize

Find a comfortable place to sit— maybe put your feet up—and think about how much time you've had during the past three days to do whatever you want to do. Mentally review your activities for each day, from morning 'til night. Use the Notes to Myself section below to add up your daily allotment of "free" time.

Start living in the moment, rather than planning for "someday." Enjoy one hour of free time today. Pencil it into your day planner as a date with yourself. Have a bubble bath, read a magazine, lie on the couch, look at old photo albums, light a candle, listen to music. Close the door on the world and relax.

How soon can you have an entire evening for yourself? A whole day? An uninterrupted weekend? Don't plan anything. Wait and see what you feel like doing at the moment—then do it!

Notes to Myself

How much "free" time have I actually had over the past three days? What did I do that was both relaxing and fun? What made me stop doing it?

A Leg Up: *Today:*	Exercise can work wonders over time, strengthening muscles, stabilizing joints, and increasing flexibility to reduce the pain of osteoarthritis.	🍐	👟	♡ **1**
Moving Moment: *Today:*	The key to sticking with any exercise program is to focus on frequency first. Increase the duration and intensity of your routine later.	🍐	👟	♡ **2**
Soul Provider: *Today:*	A simple cup of tea or coffee can be aroma therapy. Make time to relax. Try life in the slow lane.	🍐	👟	♡ **3**
Go with the Flow: *Today:*	Water helps relieve constipation. When you don't drink enough, your body draws on internal sources, such as your colon.	🍐	👟	♡ **4**
Incredible Edible: *Today:*	Studies show that vitamin C can lower blood pressure. Pass the oranges, please! And the bell peppers, cabbage, potatoes, strawberries ...	🍐	👟	♡ **5**
Goal Getter: *Today:*	Brushing your teeth immediately after the last meal of the day often reduces the temptation to snack.	🍐	👟	♡ **6**
Dine-o-Mite: *Today:*	Dried fruits, such as pears, raisins, apricots, or prunes, have a higher sugar concentration and more calories than the same amount of fresh fruit.	🍐	👟	♡ **7**

Beauty and the Best: Sometimes you see more clearly with your eyes closed than open.

Speak Easy

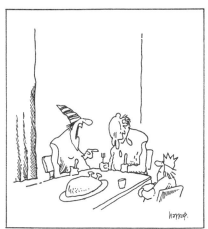

THE BOOK SAYS MEALTIMES SHOULD BE FUN — NOW CARVE THE RUBBER TURKEY...

Chat Out of the Bag

Speaking easy takes practice! Try rehearsing what you want to say by speaking into the mirror. Look yourself in the eye! Say those words you want to say—firmly, but fairly.

If speaking easy is really hard for you, consider taking a course in Assertiveness Training at your local college or community center.

Role Models

Do you admire a friend or co-worker's ability to Speak Easy without getting flustered or annoyed? Watch how she does it! Her timing. Her choice of words. Her style—does she use humor or keep a straight face?

Put Yourself in the Picture

Now and then, we all feel misunderstood. Being able to Speak Easy increases your control over everyday situations by letting others know what you think and how you feel.

Have you ever choked back the words you wanted to say and choked down cookies instead? It's not an uncommon reaction.

Many people don't speak up because they're afraid it wouldn't be "nice." They'd rather bottle up their feelings than risk losing control and exploding in anger. Occasionally they do explode, and then feel remorseful later. Practice speaking easy before resentment builds. You deserve to be heard, just like anyone else.

Speaking freely means telling someone how you feel, what you think, and what you want. It doesn't have to involve aggression, sarcasm, tears, or loud voices. The sooner you speak up in a situation, the more control you'll feel. The longer you wait, the angrier you'll get.

Speaking easy means being assertive. If someone's making "fat jokes," tell them you're uncomfortable. Others will respect you for it—and you'll respect yourself.

Herb 'n' Renewal:	Rather than use fat for flavor and texture, try crunchy barley, couscous, or whole grains seasoned with pungent spices and fragrant herbs.			**8**
Today:				
Goal Getter:	Failing to plan may mean planning to fail. Think about your food choices long before you sit at the table.			**9**
Today:				
The Light Stuff:	Raise your calcium quotient! Blenderize plain skim-milk yogurt with sliced fresh fruit and a sprinkle of skim-milk powder.			**10**
Today:				
Moving Moment:	Some of the most important benefits of exercise take place when you stop to rest, allowing muscles and tissues to repair and strengthen themselves.			**11**
Today:				
Sylph Esteem:	All foods are good foods. Junk food is less of a problem than junk food habits.			**12**
Today:				
Stats Quo:	Starting when we're in our 30s, inactivity and hormonal changes produce a lean muscle-mass loss of about half a pound (225 grams) a year.			**13**
Today:				
Soul Provider:	The best things in life aren't things, but other people.			**14**
Today:				

Beauty and the Best: As the earth turns, days become dark and nights turn to days. Life's changes are orderly rather than chaotic, complementary rather than conflicting. Accept change as a natural part of a life in balance.

Notes to Myself

How comfortable am I speaking up for myself? If I can answer "Yes!" to the following questions, I'm on track. If not, I'll follow the pointers further down on this page for a refresher course in speaking easy.

- [ ] I don't mind asking for help if I need it.
- [ ] I avoid bottling up my frustrations, correcting misunderstandings as quickly as I can.
- [ ] I let people close to me know my needs for privacy, solitude, and relaxation.
- [ ] I usually tell people what's on my mind, but I don't always expect to win them over to my point of view.
- [ ] I know how to say "no."

Design Your Plan

Review the Notes to Myself section above, taking one item from the list that you couldn't check "Yes." Make a little Speak Easy project for yourself, based on this point. Look for an opportunity to practice your new approach. If it's scary, pick an easy one first: Ask a family member to help you with a simple, pleasant task, such as shopping for vegetables at an open-air market. Ask a close friend if you can practice speaking your mind, before you approach the person with whom you'd really like to get something off your chest.

Ask yourself what could stand in your way—the feeling that speaking easy's not your style? Now think about how often you've felt frustrated because you didn't speak easy to someone. Isn't it worth a little effort to reduce that sense of helplessness and let yourself be heard?

Letting Off Steam

When a kettle lets off steam, the pressure build-up eases. When you let off steam, the same thing happens. If you simmer and don't let it out, you'll eventually get red hot and may explode. That means wear and tear on every system of your body. Over many years, it could lead to heart disease and stroke.

Cultivate Ease by allowing yourself to be heard. It's positive—and healthy!

Perfect Practice

Do you find yourself saying, "I should get more exercise. I should take more breaks. I should drink less coffee." People who do the things you think you should be doing seem like paragons of virtue! They seem so "disciplined"!

Discipline is simply training: The ultimate discipline is something you do because you want to. Because some little voice inside says, "Do it!" Take the time each day to do a little of what you like a lot. It's your life.

108

Incredible Edible: *Today:*	Substitute mashed pinto beans or black beans for half the meat in your burger. Boost fiber and flavor; trim fat.	♎	👟	♡ **15**
Soul Provider: *Today:*	Take a moment to notice the beauty around you—grass, trees, sky, clouds, stars. Consciously slow down and relax.	♎	👟	♡ **16**
Dine-o-Mite: *Today:*	Fat is essential to your diet—as long as you don't overdo it. Too little fat in your diet means brittle nails, dull, dry hair, and vitamin deficiencies.	♎	👟	♡ **17**
Stats Quo: *Today:*	More than half of us decide what to cook for dinner on the same day. Ten percent of us routinely decide at the last minute!	♎	👟	♡ **18**
Skill Power: *Today:*	It's better to make small changes consistently than large ones inconsistently.	♎	👟	♡ **19**
Moving Moment: *Today:*	Walk through airport terminals and take the stairs whenever possible. Avoid "people movers" and move yourself.	♎	👟	♡ **20**
Idle? Wild! *Today:*	Feet up! Let others wait on you! In other words, pretend you're a man.	♎	👟	♡ **21**

Beauty and the Best: The most creative people pay attention, seeing what others miss. That's why we call them visionaries.

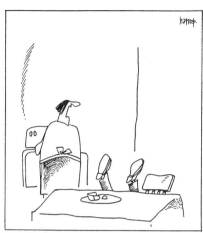

HOW'S THE IRISH WHISKEY CAKE...?

When Life Is a Cabernet

Alcohol isn't a solution to chronic stress. A glass or two may relax you at first, but alcohol can wreak havoc with your blood sugar, picking you up just to drop you down.

Admiration = Emulation

Which famous woman do you admire most? If she's written an autobiography, give it a read!

Show and Tell

Visualizations and imagery are powerful tools in every aspect of your life. Whether you "see" yourself being more assertive, exercising regularly, or eating mindfully, visualization will take you there until the image becomes reality. Use positive images that stir the senses and motivate, holding special meaning for you. There are three steps to this process:

- Visualize your goal.
- Visualize yourself with the strength and the desire to reach it.
- Visualize yourself having met your goal.

Aging Like a Fine Wine

Many women who are middle-aged today grew up with traditional notions of what it meant to be feminine: soft, gentle, quiet, passive, nurturing. But the women over 50 who are most content are those who have learned to be more assertive—while still maintaining their openness and sensitivity.

Similarly, men who "get in touch with their feminine side" seem to be more psychologically healthy than those who cling to macho stereotypes.

Studies show that women who don't develop their assertiveness, but remain as passive and dependent as they were as teenagers, worry more about aging than their more positive age-mates. Speaking up helps us feel in control—and a sense of control is a powerful determinant of health and happiness.

Binge Buster:	If you always find yourself picking at after-dinner leftovers, refrigerate them immediately or ask someone else to clean up.			22
Today:				
Just Desserts:	A single serving of sweetened yogurt may contain almost as much sugar as a regular soft drink. Read the label!			23
Today:				
Moving Moment:	Walk a friend or neighbor's dog if you don't have one of your own. It's a new leash on life!			24
Today:				
Goal Getter:	Don't wait too long to give away clothes from your former weight. Keeping them in the cupboard gives you "permission" to return to that weight.			25
Today:				
Pick Up the Pace:	Use two pairs of walking shoes rather than one. Each pair stresses the feet differently. Alternate the pairs to give your feet a treat.			26
Today:				
Go with the Flow:	Wet your whistle more often: Start each meal with water, juice, milk, or soup.			27
Today:				
Soul Provider:	Give thanks for one of the little things in your day, even if it's just finding a parking space when you need one!			28
Today:				

Beauty and the Best: Think of your food as engine fuel. Premium fuel lets your engine run lean!

Legal-Ease

Everyone—regardless of age, gender, sexual orientation, ethnic origin, religion, mental or physical challenges, or shape or size—deserves and needs respect.

Know your rights. Size discrimination is illegal in an increasing number of jurisdictions—particularly when it affects jobs or chances of promotion. Grassroots groups around the world are lobbying to add the words "size or weight" to existing anti-discrimination laws.

Cruel comments, snubs, and being made the butt of jokes can hurt your self-esteem. The Speak Easy plan will help you meet those challenges—but you may need extra support. Check your local library, community center, or the Internet to connect with size-acceptance support groups in your area.

Seek and Ye Shall Find

Healthy people have support systems. Whether friends, relatives, colleagues, or mutual-interest groups, it's important to have at least one trusted person in whom you can confide and from whom you can seek another perspective. Being isolated and alone is unhealthy. People need people.

This extends to making major lifestyle changes. Research shows that those who succeed draw on others' support. Decide what kind of support you need, and ask for it. Your needs are special. Don't assume your family and friends already know what you need. Tell them.

Top Priority

Are the people in your life your biggest priority? Ask your friends and family members what they appreciate most about you. Chances are they'll say how much fun you are to be with, how you make them laugh, how affectionate you are, how they can count on you to be there for them.

We bet dollars to doughnuts (the whole-wheat, low-fat variety, of course) that they won't say: We appreciate you because your bathroom is spotless; your table linens match your china; you drive me to piano lessons; your nail polish is never chipped; you send greeting cards early.

Watch for connections between the time you invest in activities and how much they really mean to you and yours. Did you try to do too much today? If you're too tired to enjoy it yourself, "quality" time isn't much fun for anyone else!

Stats Quo:	It takes 20 times more land to feed one person on a meat-based diet than it does to feed someone who is fully vegetarian.			**29**
Today:				

Incredible Edible:	Turn your dinner plate into a palette of vibrant colors. The darkest greens have the most beta-carotene.			**30**
Today:				

Beauty and the Best: Cherish those qualities that endure—your sense of humor, your compassion for others. Watch your changing body with wry amusement.

Put Yourself in the Picture

Last January, we talked about facing change. We admitted it can be daunting, but also said it can be exhilarating and exciting. Positive change that offers win-win solutions benefits everyone—ourselves, our families, our co-workers, our friends, as well as large groups and even nations!

Imagine for a moment the billions of health-care dollars that would be saved if everyone practiced the 3 E's of healthy living! Imagine the extra years of positive, productive living! That's the big picture—but what about your own picture?

You've been "putting yourself in the picture" these past many months. How does the picture look? Better than when you started? How does the picture feel? More like "yourself" every day? If the picture doesn't feel "right," then take another picture! You may want to adjust your goals.

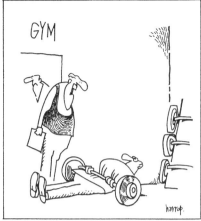

I SAID: HOW'S THE WEIGHT PROGRAM GOING ...?

See how you fare in the checklist below. Really *think* about your needs, and be upfront about them. Be firm, fair, and flexible as you choose an aspect of your support system to build on. Plan your approach and rehearse it first: Be positive! Be willing to meet others halfway.

Getting support doesn't mean losing your independence. If you like walking with a buddy, go alone some of the time to prove to yourself you can do it. It feels good to know when you need support from others and when you don't.

Notes to Myself

Can I answer "Yes!" to most of these questions? If not, I'll plan to get the support I need.

- ☐ I let people know when I need active encouragement, and when I'd rather be left alone.
- ☐ I ask for family cooperation in adjusting meal schedules so I can exercise.
- ☐ I ask for help with household chores.
- ☐ I ask people not to coax me to eat or drink.
- ☐ I treat myself in ways that reinforce healthy, satisfying habits.

Goal Getter:	If work-related reading threatens to keep you from the gym, prop those papers on the stair-climber, stationary bike, or treadmill.			
Today:				**1**
Soul Provider:	You are a sensuous being. Trust, touch, time, and tenderness are yours to give and receive.			
Today:				**2**
Moving Moment:	Lap it up! It takes less time to achieve a workout of equal intensity in chest-deep water than it does on dry land.			
Today:				**3**
Stats Quo:	The average North American child watches 10,000 TV ads each year—most of them for fatty, sugary, salty foods.			
Today:				**4**
Go with the Flow:	If your doctor approves, drink plenty of water to reduce swollen feet, legs, and hands. When your body doesn't get enough fluid, it tries to preserve every drop.			
Today:				**5**
Binge Buster:	Having a small, low-fat snack before partying or dining curbs later over-indulgence.			
Today:				**6**
Second Helpings:	Don't be discouraged by plateaus in weight loss, or by "falling off" your exercise or eating plan. Keeping positive will keep you on track.			
Today:				**7**

Beauty and the Best: No one has the right to control what you do with your body. If you want to make a change, make it for yourself—not for someone else's idea of who or what you should be.

Design Your Plan

And now it's time to ask for support. Imagine how good it feels! The easy give-and-take of building support for healthy living! Sharing walks or rides to the gym. Divvying up chores. Receiving encouragement and supporting others. Why should anything stand in your way?

Ready ... set ... flow!

- When will you start your plan?
- What might interfere with it?
- How will you overcome obstacles, if any?

Check your day planner's **Ease icon** each day you purposely seek the support you need.

The Enemy Within

If you feel you're getting nowhere in seeking the support you need, do a little soul-searching. Sometimes people sabotage their own efforts, consciously or unconsciously. Could you be putting obstacles in your own path? You may want to seek some counseling.

You may also meet some roadblocks that are completely beyond your control. For whatever reason, some people may seem determined to undermine your best efforts. They're like boulders in a stream: Go with the flow and let the current surge around them. Find someone else to provide the support you need—someone you can help too, when it's *their* turn to need support!

Help Yourself!

It's healthy to help others. Volunteers benefit mentally and physically from their altruism. Give someone the satisfaction of offering *their* support to you!

Notes to Myself

How will it *feel* to ask for the support I need? How will *I* feel when I've got it?

Nothing to Lose: *Today:*	Researchers have found that most overweight people cite disproportionally activities that involve eating as pleasurable, while people in a healthy weight range cite a broad variety of activities.	🍐	👟	♡ 8
Twist and Pout: *Today:*	Forget about your hairstyle—protect your brain! Unless yours is stationary, always wear a helmet when you ride a bike.	🍐	👟	♡ 9
Stats Quo: *Today:*	People commonly put on five to seven pounds over the holiday season. Seasonal weight-gain can add up over the years, resulting in obesity.	🍐	👟	♡ 10
Goal Getter: *Today:*	The release of aromatic volatile compounds means that hot food satisfies your hunger better than cold food. You may feel fuller with less.	🍐	👟	♡ 11
Go with the Flow: *Today:*	We lose up to 12 glasses of water each day. Water replenishes your skin, helps you breathe, delivers oxygen and nutrients to your cells, and eliminates wastes.	🍐	👟	♡ 12
Dine-o-Mite: *Today:*	Some restaurants now feature low-fat, heart-smart choices. Ask for them! And don't try to clean your plate.	🍐	👟	♡ 13
Leaps and Bounds: *Today:*	Are you off your rocker? Studies show that you can continue to enlarge and strengthen your muscles right into old age.	🍐	👟	♡ 14

Beauty and the Best: Allow yourself the gift of leisure time. Time is precious—it's a non-renewable resource!

Take a Breather

The word "inspiration" has several meanings. Among them: "Breathing in, drawing air into the lungs." We need inspiration to live fully.

What makes your heart soar? Look for *fresh* inspiration every day. Ignoring its importance is like breathing stale air.

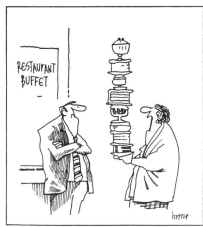

IT SAYS WE'RE ALLOWED ONE TRIP TO THE DESSERT TABLE.

- Pick up a book of poetry and read a poem aloud.
- Take a walk somewhere beautiful and really *notice* your surroundings.
- Visit a bookstore and browse in a section you've never looked at.
- Organize a magazine swap at the office.
- Occasionally trade a CD with a friend for an evening.
- Rent an acclaimed foreign film.
- Sing! Follow the words on an album cover or song sheet.
- Visit someone you admire. Ask what that person finds inspiring

Notes to Myself

Thinking back over the day, did I *respond* or *react* to situations? If "knee-jerk" reactions were the order of the day, what could I have done differently?

Binge Buster: Steamed milk with a dash of almond flavoring is a yummy substitute for eggnog. It froths up nicely if you whisk it before putting it in the microwave.

15

Today:

Sylph Esteem: Tempted by the latest "hot" supplement? Add it to a healthy diet and you'll still have a healthy diet. Add it to a poor diet and—yup!—you'll still have a poor diet.

16

Today:

Moving Moment: A Harvard University study showed that athletic swimmers in their 60s had sex as often as non-exercisers in their 40s did. Get in the swim!

17

Today:

Goal Getter: Your Eating, Exercise, and Ease choices should be pleasurable. Think of Enjoyment as the fourth "E." It's a health promoter!

18

Today:

Go with the Flow: Exercising in very cold weather can dehydrate you. Every breath you "see" contains tiny water droplets. Drink water!

19

Today:

Poultry in Motion: Sliced 'n' diced, a little bit of chicken seems like more. Serve it over veggies, rice, or a lightly tossed salad.

20

Today:

Binge Buster: We eat more in good company. Thanksgiving, Christmas/Hanukkah, and New Year's are the Bermuda Triangle of holiday feasting!

21

Today:

Beauty and the Best: You'll be less likely to seek solace in food if you believe in yourself and take responsibility for your actions. Meet life's challenges head-on!

The Art of Ease: Notes to Myself

Take a moment to review your "Easy" new habits. Focus on this week's routine.

THE ABC'S OF THE ART OF EASE:

I have:

- ☐ Adjusted my attitude.
- ☐ Become aware of my rights.
- ☐ Cared enough about my relationships to share my thoughts and needs.

Did I Pamper Myself This Week?

How Do I Feel About That?

QUICK CHECK

Breathing easy ☐ ☐ ☐ ☐ ☐ ☐

Resting easy ☐ ☐ ☐ ☐ ☐ ☐

Taking it easy ☐ ☐ ☐ ☐ ☐ ☐

Speaking easy ☐ ☐ ☐ ☐ ☐ ☐

Seeking easier ☐ ☐ ☐ ☐ ☐ ☐
solutions by
getting support

Am I on Track?

If I can answer "Yes" to most of these questions, I've boosted my Ease quotient. If not, I'll consider seeking professional advice:

- ☐ Am I starting to feel less anxious through Quieting?
- ☐ Am I experiencing fewer physical signs of stress, getting to sleep more quickly, and doing some Progressive Relaxation?
- ☐ Am I making more time for myself?
- ☐ Am I striving to be heard and saying what I feel?
- ☐ Am I more relaxed about letting others help?
- ☐ Am I creating more Ease and less guilt?
- ☐ Am I rediscovering inner joy and feeling less anger and depression?

Nothing to Lose:	List all the reasons to stay at your present size. Does your weight puff out wrinkles? Make you feel powerful? Insulate you against cold? Focus on fitness—not fatness.	🍐	👟	♡
Today:				22

Skinny Dipping:	Be a creative nibbler at holiday parties. Limit yourself to three hot appetizers and splurge on the fresh veggies.	🍐	👟	♡
Today:				23

Hello to Good Buys:	Leave Santa a memorable gift. May we suggest an exercise video, a gift certificate to a fitness center, or a book packed with healthful eating and exercise tips—like this one!	🍐	👟	♡
Today:				24

Season's Eatings:	Enjoy everything the holidays have to offer, but think about your choices. Skip the gravy and go easy on the creamed foods. A sample is usually ample!	🍐	👟	♡
Today:				25

Stats Quo:	Ten minutes of passionate sex burns 45 calories in women and 60 calories in men. Get physical!	🍐	👟	♡
Today:				26

Go with the Flow:	Limit alcohol to no more than one or two drinks a day, or avoid it altogether. Alcohol stimulates your appetite and is readily converted to fat.	🍐	👟	♡
Today:				27

Soul Provider:	Don't try to go it alone. Some problems need a new view. Talk them out with someone you trust to ease the strain.	🍐	👟	♡
Today:				28

Beauty and the Best: True wealth is neither money nor material possessions, but a calm faith in yourself and in a higher power.

Ease: Future Perfect?

We began the year with a message about size acceptance. We think that's an appropriate way to end it, too.

We urge you to remember that weight standards aren't cast in stone. You may be at your healthy best weight right now. Even if "the numbers" suggest otherwise, you can be healthy and fit at any size.

We also urge you to remember that no one else can tell you what you "should" weigh. It's your body and you have to feel comfortable with it and in it. Only you can make the decision to change your life and your lifestyle.

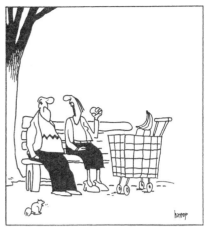

IS THIS WHAT YOU MEANT BY EATING A LA CARTE EVERY NIGHT...?

If you've already started to do that, we remind you that your new lifestyle is still evolving. Life rolls along each day, bringing fresh new challenges as it does. We also remind you that the most permanent, productive changes are those that you make for yourself —not to please someone else.

Other than feeling more active, positive, energized, and self-assertive, you may not feel that your life is very "different" than it was before. You may still have problems balancing your budget. You may still have rebellious teenagers. You may still have aging parents. But we hope you're coping better, and making more time for "you."

This lifestyle planner has not been about getting "thin." It's been about helping you reach your potential for vitality. We hope it's achieved that aim.

There is no "ideal" body size, shape, or weight. Diversity is a positive dimension of healthy living. Each of us is unique. Each of us is special. Feel good about your body and respect it. Keep this lifestyle planner as a memento of a year filled with personal growth.

Our last bit of advice: Love yourself. Few things are more important than recognizing your own worth. None of us is "perfect," but we all have something to give. Fill your days with sunshine, no matter what the weather. Be happy and be positive, but above all, be yourself. It's the best you can possibly be!

Judy and Nicole

122

Stats Quo:	In 30 percent of American households, convience is the first priority when making food decisions.	🍐	👟	♡
Today:			**29**	
Soul Provider:	Nurture your relationships. Love and support affect health more profoundly than anything else!	🍐	👟	♡
Today:			**30**	
Winner's Circle:	Celebrate your successes and forget your excesses. Happy New Year!	🍐	👟	♡
Today:			**31**	

Beauty and the Best: You must *allow* yourself to dream before your dreams can ever come true.

Acknowledgments

We thank all those who provided support, help, and inspiration along the way, especially to our husbands, Dave and David, and our children, Sarah, Erica, Roger, Samantha, and Erin.

Thank you Anna Porter, for believing in us; Clare McKeon, for listening to our verbal hand-wringing and making editing suggestions; Susan Renouf, for support and humor; and Courtenay Ireland, Debby de Groot, Bonnie Harris, Andrea Kellner, Sheila Evely, and Mary Ann McCutcheon for being so kind and helpful.

We thank the British Columbia Ministry of Health for permission to use the Physical Activity Readiness Questionnaire (PAR-Q) and the American Council on Exercise, San Diego, for use of the Perceived Exertion Rating Scale.

Our further thanks to Anne Birthistle, for creative inspiration; to Kim Stallknecht, for making our photo sessions fun; and always, to Graham Harrop, our hero and friend.

NEVER SAY DIET! FOOD CIRCLE

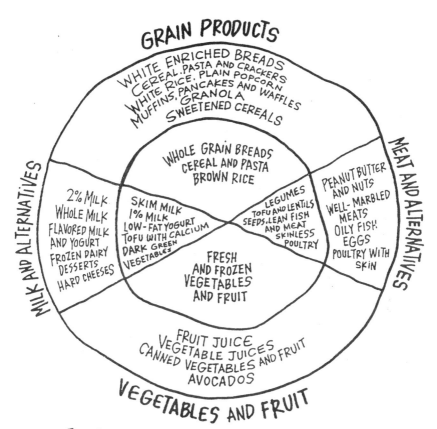

GRAIN PRODUCTS

WHITE ENRICHED BREADS
CEREAL, PASTA AND CRACKERS
WHITE RICE, PLAIN POPCORN
MUFFINS, PANCAKES AND WAFFLES
GRANOLA
SWEETENED CEREALS

WHOLE GRAIN BREADS
CEREAL AND PASTA
BROWN RICE

MILK AND ALTERNATIVES

2% MILK
WHOLE MILK
FLAVORED MILK
AND YOGURT
FROZEN DAIRY
DESSERTS
HARD CHEESES

SKIM MILK
1% MILK
LOW-FAT YOGURT
TOFU WITH CALCIUM
DARK GREEN
VEGETABLES

LEGUMES
TOFU AND LENTILS
SEEDS, LEAN FISH
AND MEAT
SKINLESS
POULTRY

MEAT AND ALTERNATIVES

PEANUT BUTTER
AND NUTS
WELL-MARBLED
MEATS
OILY FISH
EGGS
POULTRY WITH
SKIN

FRESH
AND FROZEN
VEGETABLES
AND FRUIT

FRUIT JUICE
VEGETABLE JUICES
CANNED VEGETABLES AND FRUIT
AVOCADOS

VEGETABLES AND FRUIT

OTHER FOODS INCLUDE EVERYTHING ELSE.
THERE ARE 2 TYPES:

• LOW-CALORIE/LOW-NUTRIENT ITEMS: TEA AND
COFFEE (WITHOUT CREAM AND SUGAR) AND DIET SODAS

• HIGH-CALORIE/LOW-NUTRIENT ITEMS: REGULAR SOFT
DRINKS, ALCOHOL (WINE, BEER AND SPIRITS) CANDY, CHOCOLATE BARS,
JAM, JELLY, HONEY, SUGAR, KETCHUP, LUNCHEON MEATS, BACON,
SAUSAGES, WIENERS, BUTTER, MARGARINE, OIL, SHORTENING, POTATO
CHIPS, SALAD DRESSING, MAYONNAISE, GRAVY AND ANYTHING DEEP FRIED

PAR-Q and You:
Physical Activity Readiness Questionnaire

Regular physical activity is fun and healthy, and increasingly more people are starting to become more active every day. Being more active is very safe for most people. However, some people should check with their doctor before they start becoming much more physically active.

If you are planning to become much more physically active than you are now, start by answering the seven questions in the boxes below. If you are between the ages of 15 and 69, the PAR-Q will tell you if you should check with your doctor before you start. If you are over 69 years of age, and you are not used to being very active, check with your doctor.

Common sense is your best guide when you answer these questions. Please read the questions carefully and answer each one honestly: check YES or NO.

YES	NO	
☐	☐	1. Has your doctor ever said you have a heart condition *and* that you should do only physical activity recommended by a doctor?
☐	☐	2. Do you feel chest pain when you do physical activity?
☐	☐	3. In the past month, have you had chest pain when you were not doing physical activity?
☐	☐	4. Do you lose your balance because of dizziness or do you ever lose consciousness?
☐	☐	5. Do you have a bone or joint problem that could be made worse by a change in your physical activity?
☐	☐	6. Is your doctor currently prescribing drugs (for example, water pills) for your blood pressure or heart condition?
☐	☐	7. Do you know of *any other reason* why you should not do physical activity?

If you answered YES to one or more questions, talk with your doctor by phone or in person before you start becoming much more physically active or before you have a fitness appraisal. Tell your doctor about the PAR-Q and which questions you answered YES.

- You may be able to do any activity you want—as long as you start slowly and build up gradually. Or, you may need to restrict your activities to those that are safe for you. Talk with your doctor about the kinds of activities you wish to participate in and follow his/her advice.

- Find out which community programs are safe and helpful for you.

If you answered NO honestly to all PAR-Q questions, you can be reasonably sure that you can:

- Start becoming much more physically active. Begin slowly and build up gradually. This is the safest and easiest way to go.
- Take part in a fitness appraisal. This is an excellent way to determine your basic fitness so that you can plan the best way for you to live actively.

Delay becoming much more active:

- If you are not feeling well because of a temporary illness such as a cold or a fever, wait until you feel better.
- If you are or may be pregnant, talk to your doctor before you start becoming more active.

Please note: If your health changes so that you later answer YES to any of the PAR-Q questions, tell your fitness or health professional. Ask whether you should change your physical activity plan.

Reproduced with permission from the 1994 revised version of the Physical Activity Readiness Questionnaire (PAR-Q and You). The PAR-Q and You is a copyrighted, pre-exercise screen owned by the Canadian Society for Exercise Physiology.